PENGUIN BOOKS

ENDOMETRIOSIS

Suzie Hayman trained as a teacher at Newcastle University. In 1975 she joined the Family Planning Association as press assistant, subsequently becoming press officer. She was information officer for Brook Advisory Centres from 1976 to 1984 and since then has been a freelance journalist and broadcaster. She is now a member of the National Council of the Family Planning Association and a Board member of Brook Advisory Centres. Suzie Hayman has written for national magazines such as *Woman, Woman and Home, Living, Good Housekeeping, Just 17, 19, Bella* and *Country Living*, as well as for the *Guardian* and *Sunday Times* newspapers, and is 'agony aunt' for *Essentials* magazine. She has produced educational material for the Family Planning Association, and is the author of *Hysterectomy, It's More than Sex: A Survival Guide to the Teenage Years, Living With A Teenager* and *Vasectomy and Sterilization*. She is the author of *The Well Woman Handbook*, published by Penguin in 1989. She is a frequent contributor to television and radio, and lives in Cumbria with her partner and two cats.

■ SUZIE HAYMAN

Endometriosis

Illustrated by Audrey Besterman

PENGUIN BOOKS

PENGUIN BOOKS

Published by the Penguin Group
Penguin Books Ltd, 27 Wrights Lane, London w8 5tz, England
Viking Penguin, a division of Penguin Books USA Inc.
375 Hudson Street, New York, New York 10014, USA
Penguin Books Australia Ltd, Ringwood, Victoria, Australia
Penguin Books Canada Ltd, 2801 John Street, Markham, Ontario, Canada l3r 1b4
Penguin Books (NZ) Ltd, 182–190 Wairau Road, Auckland 10, New Zealand

Penguin Books Ltd, Registered Offices: Harmondsworth, Middlesex, England

Published in Penguin Books 1991
10 9 8 7 6 5 4 3 2 1

Copyright © Suzie Hayman, 1991
Illustrations copyright © Audrey Besterman, 1991
All rights reserved

The moral right of the author has been asserted
The moral right of the illustrator has been asserted

Printed and bound in England by Clays Ltd, St Ives plc
Filmset in 10½/13 pts Ehrhardt

Contents

Acknowledgements

Many thanks for papers, information, advice, encouragement and/or suggestions to Toni Belfield, Michael Brush, Barbara Gill, Chris Glynn, Stephen Kennedy and Chris Sutton. And a very special thanks to Robin Ballard, who wields a red pen with as much precision, skill and care as he does a scalpel.

Thanks to all the women – fellow-patients, members of self-help groups, friends of friends and acquaintances (it's *amazing* once you mention this condition how many people turn out to have it!) and to those who had written to my agony page who allowed me to interview them and gave permission for their stories and words to be used to show fellow-sufferers what can happen and what can be done when you have endometriosis.

And to Vic, who having just recovered from dealing with the heartache and the thousand natural shocks that woman's flesh is heir to, had to go through yet another couvade in this one.

Introduction

Endometriosis was first described in 1860 by an Austrian doctor, von Rokitansky. He called it adenomyoma – a kind of tumour made up of muscle tissue and cells usually found in the lining of the womb, which he had found inside the walls of the womb and on the ligaments that support it. Over the next sixty years, only twenty-one other cases were described in medical literature. Then in 1924 an American doctor, J. A. Sampson, published a series of articles in various surgical and gynaecological journals detailing his findings and arousing intense academic interest in this condition, which he called endometriosis.

In the 130 years since it was first described and the three-quarters of a century since it was first subjected to detailed research, endometriosis has remained a strange and puzzling disease. Except in a very few exceptionally rare cases it affects only women, and appears not to be life-threatening – perhaps two important reasons to explain why it has not been researched as thoroughly as many other conditions, and is still under-diagnosed.

Another reason for our lack of information could be that endometriosis is, in fact, a 'new' disease. Although cases undoubtedly existed before von Rokitansky described it and Sampson investigated further, endometriosis could be a disease that has really only had a chance to become widespread in this century. The development of endometriosis is linked to the menstrual cycle, and women from earlier generations had fewer menstrual periods than we do now. Our great-grandmothers had their first period – the menarche – later, and experienced their last – the menopause – earlier than today's female. In between, regular pregnancies and breastfeeding meant that they might only have about thirty-five menstrual bleeds in a lifetime. A present-day young woman in the West will have her first period at around twelve, her last at around fifty, and only two pregnancies by the menopause. She will have gone through some 400 uninterrupted menstrual cycles, giving endometriosis ample opportunities to develop, as will be explained later in the book.

Doctors often refer to endometriosis as an 'enigmatic disease' – one that has so far defied our efforts to explain or understand, or to guarantee a full cure. They also often call it 'the disease of theories', because there are literally dozens of attempts to explain how it develops and why it arises, none of which is conclusively proven. Although we know endometriosis can give rise to symptoms such as painful periods, uncomfortable sex and infertility, we are a long way from establishing a complete and definitive list of symptoms. Nor do we have a foolproof test to diagnose the condition. The result of this is that we do not really know how many people suffer from endometriosis. We can make some informed guesses, and some researchers suggest that 1 to 2 per cent of the general female population may suffer from the condition – either diagnosed or hidden.

In the USA, it is the most common gynaecological problem requiring hospital treatment for women aged fifteen to forty-four. In the UK, it is the second most common after uterine fibroids. However, endometriosis is often present in a woman without being diagnosed. This is either because her doctors have not been able to find the cause of any problems she has been having, or because her endometriosis has not yet given rise to sufficient troublesome symptoms to warrant her seeking medical assistance in the first place. In some studies, around 10 to 25 per cent of women undergoing exploratory gynaecological operations or pelvic operations for other reasons such as sterilization were found to have endometriosis. Up to 30 per cent of women with fertility problems are found to be suffering from the condition.

The conservative estimate of one to two women in every hundred being sufferers is alarming enough, but there is much to support the theory that endometriosis is even more widespread than that. Consider the fact that over 67 per cent of the female population, about 15 million women in the UK, suffer period pain – a prime symptom of endometriosis – at some time in their lives. This is not a trivial problem. Each month, about 600,000 girls and women in the UK are forced to take time off from work or studies because of painful periods. Another 2 million or so report that they are unable to carry out normal housework at this time in the month.

In the past, painful periods were often blamed by doctors on the sufferer's 'inability to come to terms with her femininity'. Indeed, some old-fashioned doctors will still give this as the explanation and will tell their patients that the problem will clear up 'as soon as you have a baby'. Period pain for which no underlying disease can be found is called primary dysmenorrhoea, and it *does* often improve after a pregnancy. For reasons that will be discussed later, endometriosis can also improve after a pregnancy, and it is very easy to create a medical syllogism here – a logical argument which arrives at a conclusion by combining two related statements. However, a good argument *can* be made for many, if not all, cases of primary dysmenorrhoea actually being endometriosis. This mysterious disease would in this case be afflicting far more than 1 to 2 per cent of the female population and possibly even more than the higher estimates of 10 to 25 per cent. Could a major part of the female population, in fact, have or be at risk of developing endometriosis? And if so, how could this affect us, and what are we able to do about it?

This book is for any woman who has period problems, or any of the other symptoms that we will be discussing. The information and suggestions herein may be helpful if you have not yet been able to discover an adequate explanation or a cure. If you already wonder whether endometriosis might be the root cause, or will soon be considering the possibility, this may help you find out. Obviously, a book on its own cannot promise to give either a foolproof diagnosis or a cure. However, the more you know, the more likely you are to be able to obtain a proper diagnosis and a treatment plan from your medical advisers.

This book is also addressed to all women who *do* have endometriosis and their families. The aim is to help you understand as much as is already known about the disease and to give you the background and the confidence to get new information as it becomes available. The more you know, the less helpless you will be. The more confidence you have about yourself, the better you are likely to feel. And the more in control you are of the illness and its progression, treatment and management, the more chances you have of a successful outcome.

For the woman who suffers the effects of endometriosis and her family, there are few certainties. Certainly endometriosis can cause pain, discomfort, confusion and distress. Certainly, it can also puzzle, alienate and possibly anger the doctors who are struggling to find a cause for her symptoms or a cure for such a difficult condition. Family and friends trying to cope with the problems that result from the disease can also often find it difficult to offer the understanding, love and support that an endometriosis sufferer so desperately needs.

This book will try to explain what endometriosis is, why it occurs and develops, how it can affect you and how it may be treated or managed. We will look at the facts and the feelings that are involved in this most puzzling of medical conditions. For a non-fatal disease, endometriosis can have some pretty devastating effects on the quality of life of individuals and their families. Endometriosis is a disease that can strike women in the most vulnerable areas of their lives, and for this reason can be a profoundly frightening and depressing condition to have. Understanding what is going on and what you and your medical advisers can do about it can give you a flying start in fighting back.

CHAPTER ONE

What is Endometriosis?

I'd never heard of endometriosis before I was diagnosed as having it. Just the name was enough to send me into a panic. It sounded so *serious*. I came out of the consulting room in a black depression, and it was only when I saw my own doctor a few days later that I started to calm down. He went over it again, and explained the whole thing to me. The hospital doctor also had done this, but I was just so upset by the sound of it all that I went into a daze. The worst thing about having endometriosis is that nobody I know has ever heard of it. When people ask me what is wrong, I have to go into a long explanation and I can just see them thinking 'cancer', or something. I get very frightened and depressed all over again, so now I just change the subject.

What is endometriosis?

Like most medical terms, the word comes from the Greek and, when broken down into sections, explains itself. '*Endo*' means inside, and '*metra*' is uterus, or womb. Thus, 'endometrium' means 'inside of the womb'. This is the name given to the special coat of tissue that lines the uterus. When we add 'osis' on to the end of a word, we describe a disease or problem, and often mean that some abnormal increase is going on. This is exactly what happens in endometriosis.

Endometriosis is a condition in which tissue that is normally found lining the womb, grows outside the uterus. The lining of the womb – the endometrium – has a particular job to do when it grows in the right place. However, when endometrial cells are found in other areas, they can cause a range of symptoms and difficulties. To understand what happens and why, we need to consider how the female body is made and how the menstrual cycle works.

What does the female reproductive system look like, and how does it work?

Inside your body, protected by your pelvic bones, lie your reproductive organs. These are the parts of your body that are involved in sexual activity and pregnancy. At the centre is the uterus, or womb. Since the uterus has to be able to stretch to accommodate a full-sized baby and its protective fluid, many women think of it as a large, hollow bag. In fact, it is normally about the size and shape of a pear. The uterus hangs upside down with the stem end pointing downwards and backwards towards your buttocks, and the top end pointing up towards the navel. If you clench your fist, hold it just below your navel and imagine moving your hand backwards into your body, you have the site usually occupied by the uterus. It does not actually hang, high and dry, in an empty space, however. It is jostled or cushioned by all the other essential organs sheltering in the pelvic cavity. Above and around the uterus lie the coils of your bowel and the final part of your waste, or back passage, the rectum. Below is the sex and birth passage, the vagina. And below the front wall of the uterus lie the bladder and the water passage, the urethra.

The uterus is covered by a thin rubbery coat called the peritoneum, which also lines the entire body cavity that contains your reproductive organs. The walls of the uterus are some 1 to 2 cm thick. They contain blood and lymph vessels, nerves and muscles. One band of muscles runs up the front of the uterus, over the top, and back down to the cervix. These are the muscles that move during labour to force the baby out. They also contract during menstruation, to push out the blood, fluid and tissue fragments that make up the menstrual flow, and during orgasm. Scattered throughout these muscular walls are other tiny muscles. Their job is to regulate your periods. Just before your period, they respond to chemical signals by shutting off small blood

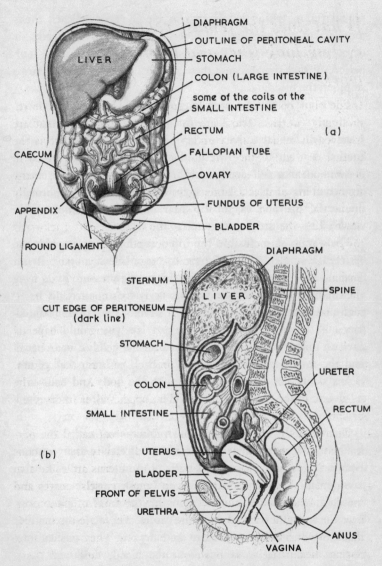

DIAPHRAGM
OUTLINE OF PERITONEAL CAVITY
STOMACH
COLON (LARGE INTESTINE)
some of the coils of the SMALL INTESTINE
RECTUM
FALLOPIAN TUBE
OVARY
FUNDUS OF UTERUS
BLADDER
LIVER
CAECUM
APPENDIX
ROUND LIGAMENT
(a)

DIAPHRAGM
STERNUM
CUT EDGE OF PERITONEUM (dark line)
STOMACH
COLON
SMALL INTESTINE
UTERUS
BLADDER
FRONT OF PELVIS
URETHRA
LIVER
SPINE
URETER
RECTUM
ANUS
VAGINA
(b)

The pelvic reproductive organs *(a) from the front, and (b) from the left side.*

vessels that lead to the next layer, the endometrium. The endometrium lines the entire uterine, or womb, cavity. It is a soft,

3

pink layer of tissue that is rich in blood vessels. When these muscles cut off the supply of blood, the endometrium begins to decay and come away as the menstrual flow. At the end of your period, further signals cause these muscles to contract even more, stopping the bleeding.

The cavity is about 3.5 cm long and the outside measurement of the part of the uterus held inside the pelvic cavity is around 5 cm long. The stem end, or cervix, or neck of the womb, adds another 2.5 cm to the length of the organ. The cervix itself projects out into the vagina, and this provides one anchor tethering the uterus in place. The os, the channel that passes through the cervix, provides one of the three openings in or out of the uterus. This channel goes through to the vagina.

The vagina is a flexible tube that reaches from its opening between a woman's legs to some 10 cm inside her body. In its normal state, this tube is squashed flat by the pressure of its own muscular walls and by the various organs that surround it. It passes into the body, but not up in a straight line. If you wanted to visualize exactly where your vagina lay, you would have to draw an imaginary line from its opening in the vulva, or external genitals, towards the small of your back. The lower wall of the vagina slants some 7 to 10 cm through the body and ends in a cul-de-sac called the vaginal vault. The upper wall is interrupted some 6 to 8 cm inside by the lump of flesh that is the cervix, with its channel to the uterus, jutting down into the vagina.

The vagina is extremely flexible, able to stretch to easily accommodate fingers, a tampon, or a penis, and to relax to let a baby pass down its length. Its narrowest and most sensitive part is the few centimetres nearest the exit to the vulva. The upper two-thirds nearest the vaginal vault are wider and far less sensitive, which is why a tampon is almost unnoticeable when pushed into place . . . and penis size really *doesn't* matter in lovemaking!

At the top end of its upside-down pear shape, the cavity of the uterus widens out and opens into two tubes – the Fallopian tubes. These reach out for some 10 to 16 cm, curving forwards to hover round the ovaries, or egg cases. Each Fallopian tube ends in finger-like projections called fimbria, which come closer to each ovary as ovulation, or egg release, approaches. The ovaries themselves are the size and shape of unshelled almonds – around 2 cm wide and 3.5 cm long. The ovaries, although often called 'egg cases', do not really contain eggs as such. What they have is thousands of immature cells that *could* grow into an ovum, or egg, if given the correct stimulus. When you were born, your ovaries actually carried up to 100,000 of such potential cells and, by the time puberty arrived, some 30,000 still remained. More than enough for the average lifetime! In fact, a modern woman having regular menstrual cycles might allow some 400 of these cells to develop into ova during her fertile years. At the menopause no ova remain.

As well as being tethered by the cervix projecting through the pelvic wall into the vagina, the uterus is held by ligaments, or bands of strong tissue. These are slung across the pelvic cavity from the pelvic walls, the bladder and the rectum. The uterus, the Fallopian tubes and the ovaries are all attached to these ligaments. However, none of the pelvic organs are, or should be, stuck firmly in one place. The uterus is supposed to be able to shift around, pivoting around the cervix. When you stand up, the uterus will be almost horizontal as long as your bladder is empty. If your bladder is full, it will push the uterus upwards and backwards. A full rectum will squash it downwards and forwards.

The first sign of puberty is usually a sudden increase in height, closely followed by the development of breasts. Hips and thighs will gain a padding of fat and the face may become fuller. The skin may become rougher in texture and downy hair will become more noticeable and darker around the genitals, under the arms and on the arms and legs. Some two years after the 'growth spurt', periods will begin.

The beginning of her periods is probably a watershed for any woman who is going to suffer endometriosis. No cases have been found *before* menarche, and very few are found after the menopause. To all intents and purposes, endometriosis is a disease entirely shackled to the menstrual cycle. More precisely, it is a

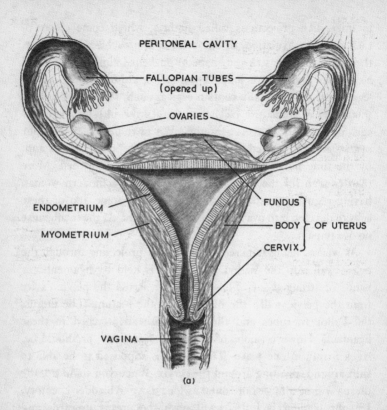

PERITONEAL CAVITY

FALLOPIAN TUBES
(opened up)

OVARIES

ENDOMETRIUM

MYOMETRIUM

FUNDUS
BODY } OF UTERUS
CERVIX

VAGINA

(a)

disease caused by one of the hormones that plays a major part in every woman's menstrual cycle and reproductive capacity. Hormones are substances produced by glands in the body that act as chemical messengers, stimulating changes or affecting various parts of the system.

The menstrual cycle starts in a small gland that is located in the base of the brain. At puberty, this begins to manufacture and release into the bloodstream a variety of chemical messengers – hormones. The hormones' first job is to trigger the gradual change from a child's body to that of a mature woman. One of these changes will be the establishing of regular monthly bleeds and of ovulation – the production every month of a potentially fertile egg. Once started, this gland then controls and regulates periods each month.

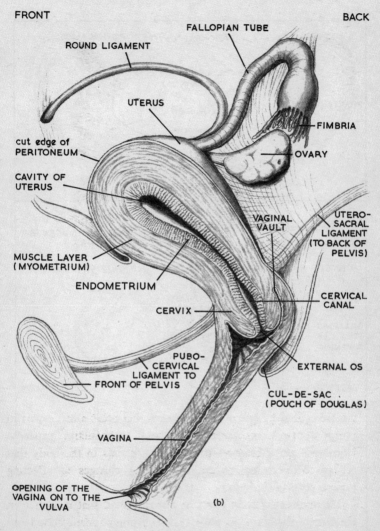

FRONT

BACK

FALLOPIAN TUBE

ROUND LIGAMENT

UTERUS

FIMBRIA

cut edge of
PERITONEUM

OVARY

CAVITY OF
UTERUS

VAGINAL
VAULT

UTERO-
SACRAL
LIGAMENT
(TO BACK OF
PELVIS)

MUSCLE LAYER
(MYOMETRIUM)

ENDOMETRIUM

CERVICAL
CANAL

CERVIX

PUBO-
CERVICAL
LIGAMENT TO
FRONT OF PELVIS

EXTERNAL OS

CUL-DE-SAC
(POUCH OF DOUGLAS)

VAGINA

OPENING OF THE
VAGINA ON TO THE
VULVA

(b)

The peritoneal cavity *(a) from the front and (b) from the left side*

The gland is called the pituitary, and is itself controlled by a part of the fore-brain called the hypothalamus. The hypothalamus is the regulator. It produces hormone-releasing agents which are chemicals that stimulate the pituitary to produce its own hormones in turn. It is worth noting that the hypothalamus has a

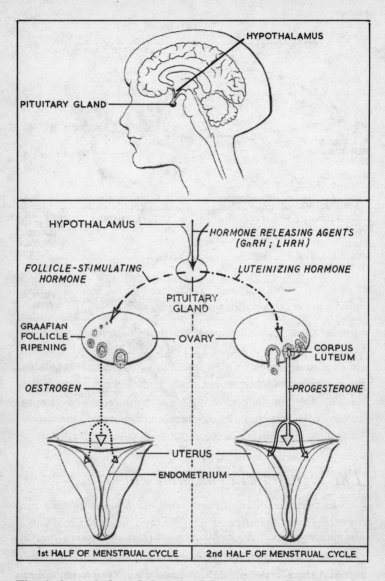

The pituitary, the hypothalamus and the pathways of hormone production

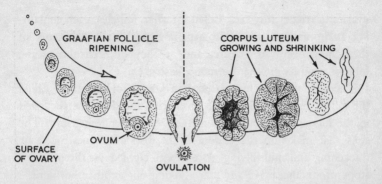

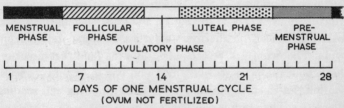

DAYS OF ONE MENSTRUAL CYCLE
(OVUM NOT FERTILIZED)

Activity in the ovary during the menstrual cycle

complex 'feedback' relationship between mind and body. It can be affected by both a woman's emotions and her physical state. If either is under stress, the hypothalamus may react by reducing the production of releasing agents, and this has the effect of shutting down or disrupting her whole hormone system. Periods may stop, become irregular or increase in flow or occurrence, and the woman may find it difficult to start or sustain a pregnancy.

The menstrual cycle and how it works

For the purposes of explanation, you will need to imagine each menstrual cycle as lasting 28 days – Day 1 being the first day of bleeding, and Day 28 being the day before the next period. In practice, your menstrual cycles can vary from 21 to 35 days, although the average is 25 to 30 days. The first five days of the cycle are called the menstrual phase. Under stimulus from the hypothalamus, the pituitary begins each menstrual cycle by producing follicle-stimulating hormone (FSH). This acts on the

9

ovaries to trigger tiny sacs, called Graafian follicles, each containing an immature ovum, into ripening. Some ten to twenty of these may begin to mature, and as they do, cells lining the follicles produce another hormone, oestrogen.

The next phase, which lasts from Day 6 to Day 12, is called the follicular phase. Oestrogen levels rise, the hormone is carried in the bloodstream and, in turn, acts on the endometrium. The cells that make up the endometrium respond to oestrogen by thickening and multiplying. After six to eight days, the pituitary stops producing FSH and starts giving out another hormone – luteinizing hormone (LH). This triggers the ovulatory phase, which lasts from Day 13 to Day 15, and causes one of the several maturing follicles on the ovary's surface to burst, releasing an ovum. The ovum will be catapulted into the fluid that circulates throughout the pelvic cavity. In around one in 117 pregnancies, two follicles ripen at the same time, both rupturing and sending out an egg. The result is non-identical twins.

At the time of ovulation, the open ends of the Fallopian tubes will have moved closer to the ovaries, and be hovering over them, ready to catch the released ovum. The Fallopian tubes are lined with hair-like protrusions, called cilia, that move and wave, setting up a current which draws the fluid from the pelvic cavity into the tubes. This wafts the newly released egg down one of the tubes and into the uterus.

Meanwhile, the luteal phase, which lasts from Day 16 to Day 23, will have begun. The site of the ruptured follicle begins its own hormone production. The ruptured area, now called the corpus luteum, begins to manufacture progesterone. This has the effect of preventing any more follicles from maturing and ripening, and of enriching and priming the endometrium to make it ready to receive a fertilized egg. The endometrium becomes thicker. The ovum takes seven to eight days to travel down the Fallopian tube from the ovary to the uterus. If conception is to take place, it must meet sufficient vigorous and live sperm in the 12 to 24 hours after ovulation before it begins to decay.

If the egg *is* fertilized it in turn secretes another hormone into

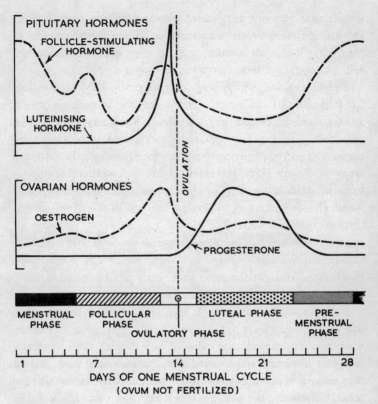

PITUITARY HORMONES
FOLLICLE-STIMULATING HORMONE
LUTEINISING HORMONE

OVULATION

OVARIAN HORMONES
OESTROGEN
PROGESTERONE

MENSTRUAL PHASE   FOLLICULAR PHASE   LUTEAL PHASE   PRE-MENSTRUAL PHASE
OVULATORY PHASE

1   7   14   21   28
DAYS OF ONE MENSTRUAL CYCLE
(OVUM NOT FERTILIZED)

The rise and fall of pituitary and ovarian hormones during the menstrual cycle

the bloodstream. This is human chorionic gonadotrophin (HCG). HCG stimulates the corpus luteum to continue producing progesterone, further encouraging the endometrium to enrich itself. If, however, the egg is not fertilized and no HCG is produced, the corpus luteum breaks down after seven days and progesterone stops being produced.

The premenstrual phase, from Day 24 to Day 28, begins with levels of oestrogen and progesterone falling sharply. After a further week, when progesterone levels have dropped, tiny muscles inside the walls of the uterus close up and cut off the blood supply to the endometrium. The lining of the womb then falls

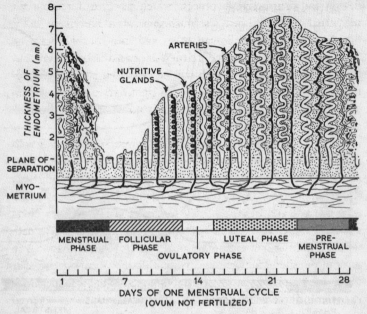

The changes in the endometrium during the menstrual cycle

away as a period – a flow of blood, tissue and fluid. As this happens, FSH levels start to pick up again and the whole cycle repeats itself.

The endometrium, then, is a constantly changing part of the body. It has the specific role to provide a welcoming environment for a fertilized egg. Endometrial cells proliferate – that is, increase and thicken – throughout the first half of the menstrual cycle, under the influence of oestrogen. Without a sufficient level of this hormone, the endometrial cells do not begin their task of growing. After ovulation, the increase in levels of progesterone make the lining even thicker and richer in blood vessels, secreting nutrients that could support a fertilized egg. The lining is called secretory endometrium at this stage. When the endometrium sloughs away, it drains from the uterus out through the os, and exits from the body through the vagina.

The uterus itself responds to changes in hormonal levels by

flexing and contracting, a process which serves to force out the menstrual contents. It can also push some blood and tissue *up* the uterus, through the Fallopian tubes and into the pelvic cavity. This phenomenon is called retrograde menstruation, and may have a significant effect which will be discussed later. The shedding process can take between two to eight days, and the amount of fluid and tissue lost may vary from individual to individual, and from period to period.

What, then, is endometriosis? This condition occurs when cells resembling endometrial tissue are found *outside* the womb. They respond to the rise and fall of hormones in exactly the same way as the endometrial tissue *inside* the womb. That is, each month cells increase and build up, only to shed and fall away as blood and fluid. When this occurs inside the womb, there is a clear path for the resulting flow to run out of the body. When it happens in most of the sites where endometriosis is found, it cannot properly drain away and that is when trouble starts. When found *outside* the womb, these cells resembling endometrial tissue are referred to as endometriotic tissue.

Where is endometriosis found?

Patches of endometriotic tissue are usually found in the peritoneal area – that is, the space in the body in which the stomach, spleen, liver, intestines, rectum, bladder, uterus and ovaries are found. The patches occur mostly in the lower portion, within the pelvis. Common sites are on the ovaries, the various ligaments that hold the uterus in place and the culs-de-sac, or pouches, such as the pouch of Douglas. Cul-de-sacs are formed when the covering of the peritoneal cavity (the peritoneum) sweeps down an organ – in this case, the uterus – and does a U-turn to travel up another organ or the wall of the pelvis – in this case, the rectum.

Endometriotic tissue is also found on the peritoneum at any point around the pelvic cavity and on the Fallopian tubes, the outside of the uterus, the cervix, the walls of the vagina, the bladder, the bowel and on the water passage, or urethra. It can also be found at sites quite removed from the reproductive organs – in lung tissue, in the sigmoid colon, in the caecum (the pouch at the end of the small intestine), in the appendix, in the soft tissue inside the nose and in sites outside the body. Externally, the tissue can be found on the vulva or outer genitals, and on the perineal body – the area of skin that lies between the vagina and the anus, or back passage.

Endometriosis has a particular affinity for scar tissue and often appears where there are healed operation wounds, as well as in the umbilicus, or navel. Very rarely, endometriosis has been found in the breast, pancreas and liver. Patches of tissue can occur on the surface of all these sites, or inside them in the tissue itself.

What does endometriosis look like?

If you were to look at an infected area, you might see several signs. These would depend on the site, and on how long the condition had been going on. You may see a lesion or damaged area on the surface which can look brownish. These are often called 'powder burn' lesions as they look as if the area has been marked with a scattering of dark burns from the back-fire of an old-fashioned gun.

Sometimes, the area is raised and reddish or reddish-blue. During your period, of course, these areas would leak fresh blood. Areas of endometriosis then form into cysts, especially if the patch has started inside rather than on the surface of the tissue. Fluid that has been unable to drain away collects inside a fibrous wall, and each bleed makes the cyst grow bigger. As time passes, the contained blood degrades. Such cysts are often called 'chocolate' cysts because the contents look like liquid chocolate. Recent bleeding makes the fluid inside the cysts have a more red or chocolate-brown appearance and a syrupy, tar-like consistency. As they get older, the cysts can look blue or have a yellow or straw colour, and sometimes the liquid becomes clear.

After a time, these patches of endometriotic tissue will become surrounded by 'fibrous adhesions'. The surface of the organs that

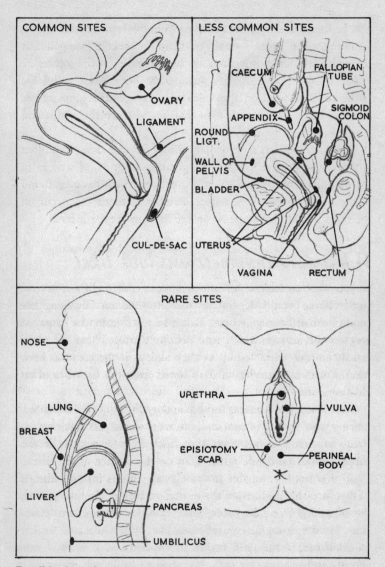

Possible sites of endometriosis

come into contact with the blood, either fresh or decaying, will react, since blood is a highly irritant substance in the wrong place and at the wrong time. The surrounding area can become quite

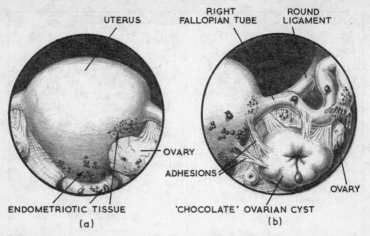

UTERUS

RIGHT
FALLOPIAN TUBE

ROUND
LIGAMENT

OVARY

ADHESIONS

OVARY

ENDOMETRIOTIC TISSUE
(a)

'CHOCOLATE' OVARIAN CYST
(b)

What endometriotic tissue looks like seen through a laparoscope
(a) mild and (b) severe

inflamed. Scar tissue will form and, if the disease continues unchecked, the areas of scar tissue can become dense. These areas form adhesions, when patches of scarring extend from one organ to another, enlarging and sticking them together. This may create an obstruction and prevent an organ carrying out its function. For instance, adhesions can stick coils of the bowel together, so they cannot expand to their full width in order to pass waste matter along the passage; the Fallopian tubes may be adhered in such a way that the open end cannot move nearer the ovary at ovulation; or, the ligaments that hold the uterus may become firmly stuck to the wall of the pelvic cavity.

The condition we call endometriosis really has two aspects. These are the patches of tissue that resemble the lining of the womb and grow in the wrong place; and the *effect* of having such tissue in the wrong place – inflammation, cysts and scar tissue.

As already mentioned, organs in the body, such as the bowel, uterus and ovaries, are only supposed to be loosely tethered in place and should have quite a degree of flexibility. Scar tissue and adhesions can give rise to very unpleasant symptoms. What these may be and how they could affect you will be discussed in Chapter 3.

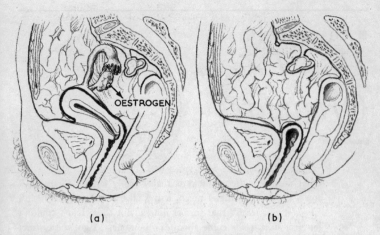

The effects of hysterectomy and oophorectomy *(a) before operation, and (b) after hysterectomy and bilateral salpingo oophorectomy*

Before we look at the possible results of having endometrial tissue growing outside the womb, however, you might like to consider the next logical question that usually arises.

> My doctor told me I had this disease, but I just couldn't get it straight how I could have caught it. It seemed that every time I asked, I was told something different and I couldn't work out whether I'd done something that gave it to me, or had it off my husband, or got it from the family.

Some of the theories about the causes of endometriosis are the subject of the next chapter.

■ CHAPTER TWO

How Endometriosis Originates

___

> What mostly bothered me was that I really couldn't figure out how I'd got this thing. I mean, it was all explained that I hadn't *caught* it – it wasn't that sort of illness. But then, I just couldn't get clear how it *had* come about. To be honest, I got the distinct impression after a time that the reason I couldn't understand all about it from my own doctor was that he wasn't all that clear himself!

There are several theories to explain how and why endometriosis occurs. Before we look at the main ones, it is worth eliminating some of the things that do *not* cause the condition. Endometriosis is still considered by some doctors to be a disease of the white, middle-aged, middle-class woman. It is, in fact, often still referred to as the 'career woman's disease'. Of course, the problem with a label such as this is that it serves as a red herring, deflecting some doctors from the proper trail.

> I know that when my GP saw me after getting a report from the hospital gynaecologist, he apologized for not having spotted the disease himself. He said, 'Of course, I should have realized your problem is endometriosis. Career women do get this a lot,' as if that should make me feel better. I don't *want* to be a career woman – it sounds so cold and calculating. I want to be a mother, and it's only this filthy disease that stops me being one. I've put everything into my job because I haven't got a choice, and I felt like crying when he said that.
>
> I had an operation because I'd been having period pains for years, and my doctor kept saying I'd grow out of it. Well, I'd obviously been having this problem for a long time because I had big cysts, adhesions and what have you. When I saw my own

doctor again, she was almost annoyed with me. She kept telling me that young people don't get this, which is why she hadn't known what it was. It was almost as if it was my fault for being different, so that it wouldn't be her fault for being wrong.

The myths about endometriosis

Until fairly recently, endometriosis *was* most often diagnosed in professional, childless women in their thirties, but this has served to erect certain myths about the condition, all of which can delay diagnosis and treatment and put an unfair burden on the sufferer. Myths such as:

1. It is an illness only found in white career women in their thirties.
2. It is stress-related.
3. Certain methods of contraception, particularly the IUD, increase the risks of developing it.
4. It is caused when women delay childbearing.

As with most myths, there is a certain element of fact in some of these statements, which serves to justify the rest. However, the main result is to throw the burden of having the disease back on the woman. In effect, they say, 'The disease is your *fault*. If you hadn't used contraception and avoided being a proper woman; if you hadn't been so unnatural as to pursue a career instead of staying home where you belonged, you wouldn't be in this position now.' It can also mean that if you turn up in front of your doctor with many of the symptoms of the disease but falling *outside* the category of patient he or she might *expect* to suffer endometriosis, your doctor might simply not think of this condition in trying to work out what is wrong with you. However, is there any truth in these beliefs?

AGE, STATUS AND RACE

Certainly, endometriosis has been a disease most often *found* in the professional woman in her thirties. But there is growing evidence to show that this does not reflect the pattern of the disease, but of diagnosis. It is more a reflection of the willingness or the ability of the doctors to diagnose it in this section of the population, than proof that this and only this group suffers the disease. Black women *do* develop endometriosis, but their symptoms are sometimes dismissed as the symptoms of PID (pelvic inflammatory disease), caused by a sexually transmitted disease, by those doctors who pay more attention to the myths of black promiscuity than to their patients.

Professional, middle-aged women are also more likely to persist until a proper diagnosis is found, than is a woman from a background, or at an age, that makes it difficult for her to stand up to someone in authority. Teenagers develop endometriosis, but their symptoms can be dismissed as being a normal part of growing up. A poor adjustment to becoming a woman or a low tolerance of 'normal' discomfort are often blamed. Many women who persist and eventually obtain a proper diagnosis of the condition in their late twenties or thirties can trace the beginnings of their discomfort back to teenage years. These myths would be more than annoying if they 'just' meant that many people have had to suffer needless discomfort for so long. Advanced endometriosis, however, can cause a lot more than the occasional stomachache, as we will discuss.

> After having endometriosis for about five years, I made a real effort to read all the books, and even struggled through medical texts and papers on it. The frightening and fascinating thing was, that at forty, I could trace symptoms back to my adolescence. I've had illness and symptoms over the last twenty-five years that actually all lock together and are all part of endometriosis. But what makes me really angry is the thought that if all those times I'd been off school I hadn't just been told to pull myself together and take two aspirins, if somebody had taken me seriously and *done* something, I might not have had to have my hysterectomy.

CONTRACEPTION

Neither has endometriosis been found to have any link with the use of various methods of birth control. Some women may be frightened that they may have made themselves vulnerable by using the Pill, since it has an effect on the hormone system. Similar fears may be felt about the IUD, since it may rely for part of its contraceptive effect on irritating the lining of the womb; or the cap – or, indeed tampons – because by blocking the route that allows blood and fluid to exit from the womb, they might have increased retrograde menstruation. None of these fears has been shown to have any foundation. Indeed, the oral contraceptive Pill may well even help to give a protective effect in some cases.

STRESS

Stress is not a cause of endometriosis, and neither is being 'highly strung'. The pain and the discomfort caused by the disease, however, can result in both – and often does.

> The doctor who saw me and diagnosed me as having endometriosis gave me a long lecture on relaxing and not being so tense. He really did seem to be saying that this was all the result of my being strung up and nervous. I was so humiliated that I burst into tears. And he was so blind and *smug* that I could have killed him. I just couldn't get through to him that I wasn't like this before it all started – I *wasn't*. But I'd had pain and sickness for years, and my marriage was on the rocks, so what did he *expect*? But he couldn't see that the illness made me nervous – it wasn't the nerves that gave me endometriosis.

DELAYED CHILDBEARING

As for delayed childbearing 'causing' endometriosis, there is just as much a case for claiming that it is the disease that causes the delay; endometriosis and infertility do seem to go together. However, the connection is complex and will be discussed at length in a later chapter. Certainly, no responsible and caring doctor would ever *blame* a woman for 'giving herself' endometriosis in this way.

How does endometriosis start?

If endometriosis is a condition in which cells that are usually found lining the womb are found in other parts of the body, how do they get there? One theory to explain endometriosis is the implantation theory.

THE IMPLANTATION THEORY

This is often called Sampson's theory, after the doctor who first described endometriosis and published a number of papers in the 1920s. He suggested that endometriosis results from endometrial fragments passing up through the Fallopian tubes during menstruation and implanting in the pelvic cavity. The flow that makes up your period is a mixture of blood, fluid and tiny fragments of tissue. Many studies have confirmed what Sampson and other surgeons observed, that during a woman's period retrograde menstruation may take place.

It is certainly true that the distribution of endometriosis could support this thinking. Endometriosis tends to occur in 'dependent' sites in the pelvis, areas that might catch and hold the endometrial tissue as it is pushed out of the Fallopian tubes into the pelvis. Studies have shown that endometrial tissue 'transplanted' from its usual site *can* bed down in a new area and flourish. They have also shown that women with endometriosis are more likely to have a retroverted uterus, that is, a uterus lying with its top tipped back and the cervix jutting forwards into the vagina. Women with this condition tend to have a heavier retrograde menstrual flow.

An extension of this theory suggests that endometriosis can be 'iatrogenic', that is, caused by doctors. The condition has a liking for scar tissue and often appears in operation scars, especially in episiotomy (the cut made in the skin behind the birth passage to widen it during childbirth) or in Caesarean scars. Other gynaecological operations such as laparotomy (a cut in the lower abdomen to look into the pelvis) can lead to endometriosis in the resulting scar. The theory is that endometrial cells are carried out of the

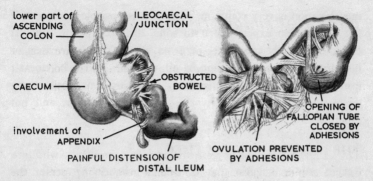

lower part of
ASCENDING
COLON

ILEOCAECAL
JUNCTION

OBSTRUCTED
BOWEL

CAECUM

involvement of
APPENDIX

PAINFUL DISTENSION OF
DISTAL ILEUM

OPENING OF
FALLOPIAN TUBE
CLOSED BY
ADHESIONS

OVULATION PREVENTED
BY ADHESIONS

The effects of adhesion

womb through bleeding or by instruments during the operation, 'seed' in the wound and continue to grow as before once the area heals. This is called the mechanical transplantation theory.

LYMPHATIC AND VASCULAR METASTASIS THEORIES

A further idea is that endometrial cells can even be carried through both blood and lymph vessels. Metastasis means the transfer of a disease or condition from one organ or part of the body to another not directly connected with it. Blood circulates throughout the body by a network of arteries and veins, carrying oxygen and nutrients. The lymphatic system runs parallel. It acts as a filter, as life-giving substances flow from the blood into the cells, and returns the remaining tissue fluid back to the blood. This would explain why endometriosis can be found in sites far away from the pelvis and in women who have not had operations. Endometriosis has been found in the liver, pancreas, gall bladder, intestine and lungs, as well as in the less distant but apparently unrelated bladder, kidneys and water passage. It has also been found in the groin and lymph nodes, in veins, and on the spine, skin and navel.

However, while these two theories explain how endometrial cells could have travelled to the sites in question, and studies show that these cells can remain viable and able to live, there are flaws in them and questions that are not answered. Retrograde menstruation is very common. In fact, it is possible that most, if not all, women experience it to some degree at some time. If endometrial cells can travel in some women's blood vessels or lymphatic systems, why not in all women? And why doesn't every woman who has an episiotomy, a Caesarean or a laparotomy develop endometriosis? Why do *some* women suffer, and not others?

THE IMMUNE SYSTEM THEORY

Recent studies suggest that in women who do *not* suffer endometriosis, endometrial cells transplanted by retrograde menstruation or any other method are attacked and disposed of by the body's own defences. Your body has a defence against invading illnesses which is called the immune response, and protects itself against bacteria with physical barriers. For example, your nose is lined with hairs and mucus membrane, to trap any large particles that try to enter which are then attacked and destroyed by killer cells produced in the mucus. Bacteria that are too small to be trapped, or that are inhaled through the mouth, are passed down the throat, swallowed and killed by the acid produced in the digestive tract or the helpful bacteria that colonize our bodies and protect us against foreign bacteria. Particles that are inhaled or that enter the body through other openings, a cut for instance, are dealt with by the body's scavenger cells.

These scavengers are called phagocytes, which means that their function is to eat or overwhelm other cells. Some phagocytes stay in one place, such as the spleen or liver, and purify the blood as it passes through these organs. Others wander about throughout the body, attacking foreign bodies where they find them. Sometimes, a disease gets through these filters and is too strong for the wandering phagocytes, so the immune system acts and produces antibodies. These are proteins which are specifically tailored to fight and overwhelm the particular invading particle.

The antibodies are produced in cells which live in the lymph tissue, and although once the attack is dealt with the level of antibody in the blood drops, the cells remember how to make them. If the same disease strikes again, the immune system can react immediately, manufacturing the precise chemicals needed to kill the invader at once. This way, having had German measles once, you will not get it again because it will be overwhelmed and stopped before you can even feel ill. This is how immunization and vaccination work – by giving you a tiny dose of the illness to allow your body to manufacture the antibodies to repel any full-blown, real invasion.

Problems come, however, if the immune system makes an error. Sometimes, it attacks the body's own cells, mistaking them for invading foreigners. Insulin-dependent diabetes, for instance, is now thought to be caused when the body's immune system attacks and kills the insulin-producing cells of the pancreas. This is called having an auto-immune disease, a condition caused by your own body destroying its own healthy cells. There is conflicting evidence to suggest that endometriosis has some associations with altered immunity. Some studies suggest that if your immune system *is* deficient in some way, even a small amount of retrograde menstruation could lead to endometriosis. Also, that heavy retrograde menstruation would overwhelm even a strong immune system's ability to deal with endometrial tissue implanting in the pelvis. Certainly, symptoms that many endometriosis sufferers report, which will be discussed in the next chapter, could suggest an auto-immune link.

THE COELOMIC METAPLASIA THEORY

A further theory to explain endometriosis is the coelomic meta-plasia theory. Metaplasia means the changing of cell tissue into an abnormal form. Coelomic cells are some of the original building blocks of the embryo. The parts of the embryo that develop into the reproductive system and the walls of the pelvis are, during the early stages of development, all the same. At that stage, they are 'undifferentiated cells' – cells capable of forming into the many various and complex cells that make up the different layers of the peritoneum, the ovaries or the uterus. This theory suggests that some of these cells remain in their original form, as undifferentiated cells without a function, and hide among other cells that have all taken on a particular job. Under some stimulus, they then suddenly change into endometrial cells and start doing the job of thickening and bleeding . . . but in the wrong place. Or, alternatively, instead of hiding as original cells without a job, they *do* spend years masquerading as ordinary cells belonging to the pelvic wall or the ovaries, and when the stimulus comes, change from these cells into endometrial ones.

This alternative theory could explain the presence of endometriosis in areas which have no easily traceable link to the pelvic cavity, such as the nose, the lungs and the skin. It would also explain why there have been three recorded cases of *men* developing endometriosis. The stimulus in their cases was in having to take long courses of oestrogen therapy to treat prostate cancer. It certainly seems that exposure to oestrogen is what stimulates endometriosis to develop. No case has yet been found in a girl before puberty – when the ovaries start to manufacture large amounts of oestrogen – and, in the main, endometriosis ceases after the menopause, when the ovaries cease to function.

Whatever the actual cause of endometriosis, there is evidence to suggest that it runs in families. The inherited factor could be an increased tendency towards auto-immune disease, retrograde menstruation, coelomic metaplasia, or a factor undiscovered as yet. But certainly studies so far seem to suggest that women whose mothers, aunts or sisters have suffered endometriosis, have an approximately 7 per cent likelihood of developing the condition too. If you accept the 1 to 2 per cent likelihood calculated for the general population, you can see that this is a noticeably increased risk.

An understanding of how and why endometriosis develops may be absolutely vital for the medical professionals if they are to help those of us who suffer from it. It may matter less to you, and what may seem more important is to understand how the disease may affect you and what can be done about it. These are the subjects of the following chapters.

■ CHAPTER THREE

Symptoms and Effects

Pain. Pain and sickness, especially just before my period.

I had this dreadful urge to go to the loo, all the time, before my period. I knew it wasn't cystitis. I'd had that, and it was different. And then I started to get a low, deep ache in my stomach at the same time, for about a week just before my period.

Passing a motion was agony. I'd get this deep ache and horrible gripping spasms as I went. Horrible.

Sex was awful. It hurt. And then I'd feel so guilty because I thought I must be doing something wrong.

Oh no, I had no pain at all, nothing. With me, it was that I couldn't fall pregnant. We had tried for three years before I went to my doctor, and I know he asked all the right questions – we remembered them afterwards. But sex was fine, my periods were fine. I just couldn't get pregnant.

I put on weight and I felt cold, tired and depressed. I was very, very low, but it was my doctor who decided I also had painful periods and that sex hurt me. I'm not stupid, but I thought that was how it was meant to be. Well, not *meant* to be, but that I was unlucky or had to put up with it.

Some illnesses are easy to recognize, both by the sufferer and the doctor. If you seemed to develop a bad cold with high fever, sore and reddened eyes which hurt in the light, a barking cough and a blotchy red rash that spreads from behind the ears over the chest and body, it wouldn't take a genius to diagnose measles. The common cold, diabetes, thyroid-gland disorders, infectious fevers . . . all tend to have an array of classic symptoms that will be either recognized by the sufferer or spotted by the doctor. But endometriosis presents difficulties, both to the woman and to the medical professionals.

Main symptoms of endometriosis

There *are* some classic signs that would suggest that your problem might be endometriosis. Dysmenorrhoea (painful periods) and dyspareunia (painful sex) are two such symptoms that may ring bells with your doctor. Menstrual problems, such as abnormal or heavy bleeding, may also suggest this diagnosis, as may a history of infertility. But women with endometriosis often have a staggeringly wide range of symptoms that may be associated with their illness. Problems can arise when a particular sufferer experiences acute discomfort from symptoms that a general practitioner might not immediately associate with endometriosis, and does *not* have any of the more obvious signs. It may help if we were to look at all the *possible* difficulties that could be present if endometriosis has developed, and understand *why* the condition gives rise to each one.

PAIN

The majority of women with endometriosis who seek help do so because they are in pain. Unfortunately, we have no way of being able to monitor pain. It is possible to look at an infected wound, a broken leg, or the results of a blood test and say, 'Yes, I can see that we have a definite problem here,' but there is no equivalent way of testing pain and saying, 'Yes, you have a reason to complain!'. We have to take the sufferer's word for it when she says that what she is experiencing is out of the ordinary and insufferable.

This, unfortunately, can mean that when we go to a doctor for help, and the main symptom we are offering is pain, we are at the mercy of the doctor's personal beliefs. If the GPs we consult feel that women often make a fuss about nothing, have a low tolerance of, or exaggerate, pain, then we may not get much help from them. A doctor who believes that pain is a subjective symptom and that if the patient *says* it is unusual and unbearable, it *is* unusual and unbearable, would offer more sympathy and practical help.

There is no doubt that different people have different reactions to the same stimulus, and what is bearable to one is not to another. This is not, however, the same as saying that some people are 'weaker' than others and should try harder to cope. Individuals will put up with more pain when their emotional and physical health is better than when they are feeling under the weather or unsupported by family, friends, or medical advisers.

Pain usually occurs just before and during periods and may be experienced as sharp spasmodic cramps. It can also occur at and around ovulation. Pain associated with endometriosis can be experienced as a constant ache, or occur only under some stimulus – when passing water, having a bowel movement, or when making love. Sometimes, the sufferer can have an idea of exactly *where* the pain is located in her body, and can point her doctor to a particular spot. With other women, the pain seems to radiate around a wide area, or to move.

Endometriosis causes pain in several ways. Firstly, the patches of endometriotic tissue may produce chemicals that cause discomfort. We now believe that dysmenorrhoea, or painful periods, is due to the lining of the uterus producing substances called prostaglandins. These encourage the uterus to flex and contract, a necessary movement during menstruation as it helps force out the menstrual blood, fluid and tissue. However, too much production of these chemicals makes the cramps become overvigorous and downright painful.

While the pain from uterine contractions cannot be assessed, the force of those movements can. Contractions during menstruation in women with a high level of prostaglandins have been found to be as strong as those in women giving birth. And, obviously, the more endometrial tissue you have, the more prostaglandins are produced. It is also possible that the endometriotic deposits may produce other chemicals that irritate the lining of the pelvic cavity. Patches of endometriotic tissue in places that can be reached by the sufferer or her sexual partner, such as the vagina, the perineum, or the vulva, may be tender to touch.

The blood and fluid leaking from endometriotic tissue can irritate surrounding tissue and this in itself causes discomfort. So too does the inevitable effect of all this irritation – scar tissue and adhesions that pull and twist the walls of the pelvis and various organs. Pelvic bodies, such as the uterus and the ovaries, become stuck to each other or to the pelvic wall, and pain can then arise if they are moved. This can happen when you move around and the organs try to flex as they would normally.

> Just before I had my operation, I was doing keep-fit. In the middle of some exercises – I think it was sit-ups or something else that meant I was using my stomach muscles strongly, moving and twisting – I felt a distinct 'tearing' sensation, and pain inside me. It wasn't agonizing, just a bit alarming and rather painful. It might have been my imagination. After all, I knew what sort of a mess I was inside so I might have been rather suggestible. But I'm sure I'd felt one of the adhesions 'go' as I moved around. I can't tell you how relieved I was that I was going into hospital the following week.

Pain can also happen when you make love, and the ligaments try to contract to pull the uterus up and out of the way. It can be a response to your own body's rising excitement, or occur when your lover penetrates you and his penis presses against the unmoving mass of adhesions inside you. Pain can also be felt when your bowel tries to move waste matter down its length with the waves of muscular contractions called peristalsis.

Why can you pinpoint some pain, and why is some vague?

The pelvis has a network of nerves that will transmit pain signals. Fibres in the skin, muscles and the peritoneum will notice inflammation or stretching, and tell you exactly where they feel discomfort. But other nerves radiate through the pelvic organs and transmit signals that are less clear. Pain felt from the crushing or distorting of some areas may be referred, or echoed, round your system, so that the pain appears to be coming from a place distant to the actual harmed area, or you cannot really tell *where* it hurts.

> Even after having my right ovary removed, I continued to get a dull, continuous ache from the same place. I no longer had a womb or Fallopian tubes, and my surgeon had spent literally hours removing every scrap of scar tissue and endometriosis he could find in the pelvic cavity. So, the only place, we later decided, it *could* be was in the top of my vagina, deep inside the wall. But that wasn't where I felt any pain. The pain was apparently distinctly coming from where my right ovary should have been and no longer was!

The curious aspect of endometriosis is that the size or age of the lesions often has very little to do with the extent of the pain they produce. There have been cases of women having exploratory operations for other reasons who have not felt any pain or had other difficulties but are found to have quite advanced scar tissue and lesions in the pelvis. Worse, there are cases of women who have complained for some time of *acute* pain whose surgeons have looked and found no evidence of any problems, but who are eventually discovered to have small endometriotic deposits.

> Over the years, I've had three exploratory operations. The doctor finally found a small patch of tissue. He told me afterwards that he still hadn't found out what had been causing my problems, but that he had found a mild case of endometriosis and removed it while he was there. To this day, I haven't had that pain again.

As yet, we just do not know enough about this disease to be able to clearly pinpoint why some cases cause more pain than others.

MENSTRUAL PROBLEMS

Apart from pain just before and during periods, endometriosis can lead to other irregular difficulties with menstruation. You may find that your periods become very erratic and either light and infrequent, very frequent indeed, or heavy and long. You may also bleed at ovulation. The blood flow itself can be unusually full of clots and be a dark brown colour. Some women report bleeding after sex, and both this and the dark flow could most likely happen when endometriosis is located in the cervix or in the vagina. The dark, tarry blood is then issuing directly from the

31

endometriotic lesions, which may also be stimulated to bleed by contact with the man's semen. One of the classic signs of endometriosis is premenstrual 'spotting'. Here, the period does not start with a sudden, regular flow, but seems to stop and start and show with spots of blood for a day or so first.

> If my period started while I was asleep, I would mostly wake up with a mild flow. But I never woke to stained sheets, and mostly what would happen is that I'd get a few spots on and off for a day or so, and then it would start properly. I can remember sharing notes with my aunt who said she used two tampons and a towel for the first two days of her periods, and then only a towel, because her flow started very heavily and then tapered off. I said I used a towel and then tampons, because mine stuttered and fiddled about and only really got going after a day. It didn't occur to me that my pattern of flow should be unusual or significant. In fact, I never mentioned it to my doctor when I did complain about period problems, and it was only brought to my attention by the hospital doctor.

The reason for these symptoms is not really clear. Endometriosis in the wall of the womb (adenomyosis) might contribute to a heavier flow in much the same way as does a uterine fibroid. By increasing the size of the womb and stretching the lining, the swelling in the uterus wall will increase the amount of endometrium *inside* the uterus and so increase the amount shed and lost at menstruation. But the exact mechanism that causes scanty or infrequent bleeds is not yet fully known.

Endometriosis can be associated with a range of difficulties with the hormonal system, and these can upset the menstrual cycle. They can also lead to the third major symptom associated with endometriosis, infertility.

INFERTILITY

Difficulty in starting or sustaining a pregnancy is often a major symptom leading to a diagnosis of endometriosis. However, the connections between endometriosis and infertility are so complex that they need to be considered in a separate chapter of their own, and we will do this later.

OTHER SYMPTOMS

Sufferers from endometriosis have reported a far wider *range* of symptoms that clearly *are* associated with the condition. Sufferers can frequently feel tired, cold, depressed or nauseous. They may complain of having pains in the joints, as well as in the pelvis, and be either frequently constipated or loose-bowelled, or, more often, swing bewilderingly between the two states. One explanation for the feelings of tiredness and general ill health which bother many endometriosis sufferers is that they may also have a degree of thyroid auto-immune disease.

Thyroid auto-immune disease

The thyroid gland is located in the throat and secretes hormones into the blood which control the speed at which the body uses oxygen and food – the metabolic rate. There are two hormones that do this, thyroxine and triiodothyronine. Thyroxine encourages cells to use up oxygen and food to produce energy, and the body to use protein and calcium to grow healthy bones and tissue. Too much thyroxine, and your body goes into overdrive and uses up stores at an unnatural rate. Your eyes may then bulge, you may feel hot and sweat heavily, feel hungry but lose weight, and have a rapid pulse and an irregular heartbeat. Not enough thyroxine, however, and you may feel tired, become forgetful, feel cold and gain weight.

One study showed that although a routine test for a thyroid condition appeared normal, the number of women with thyroid antibodies was significantly higher among endometriosis sufferers than among women not having this disease. In other words, something had caused the endometriosis sufferers' own immune systems to create antibodies to the thyroid gland, making it underactive. The amount of thyroxine available in their bodies may not have been dangerously low, but it was certainly at the lower end of the safe scale. When treated with low doses of thyroxine, their health improved.

Joint pain

It has also been suggested that some endometriosis sufferers can complain of painful joints. This is another symptom that appears to have no connection with the condition, and yet seems to occur in endometriosis sufferers more often than might have been expected in an ordinary group of women. It is worth noting that rheumatoid arthritis – one cause of pain, inflammation, stiffness and swelling in the joints – is also now thought to be an auto-immune disorder, and one that is often passed down in families.

Endometriosis in the gastro-intestinal tract

In some women, difficulties are not centred on the uterus, but on the gastro-intestinal tract – the long tube that goes down from the mouth as the oesophagus, widens to become the stomach, narrows to become the small and then large intestine before exiting the body at the anus. Endometriosis can occur in the last part of the small intestine – the ileum – and in the various parts of the large intestine – the caecum, the appendix, the sigmoid colon and the rectum. Lesions can occur on the outside of the intestine, causing adhesions which fix coils of the bowel together or attach them to the pelvic walls. Sometimes, the endometriotic tissue invades the smooth muscle layers that make up the in-testine, or even extends through to the mucous membrane that lines this tube. Adhesions can create obstructions and bleeding in the muscle layers and cause the walls to collapse in and fold on them-selves. The result may be pain and bleeding from the back passage around period times. At other times, there could be diarrhoea or constipation and possibly indigestion, nausea and vomiting.

Endometriosis in other sites

Endometriosis of the urinary tract can lead to your needing to pass water often and urgently, and can sometimes cause blood in the urine around period time. Endometriosis sufferers with urinary-tract lesions can have a feeling of 'heaviness' and pressure around the bladder.

Some endometriosis sufferers have complained of pain in the

chest area and have difficulties in breathing and either gas or liquid in the cavity around the lungs – the pleural cavity – especially just before menstruation.

Pain or tenderness around the navel or in healed operation wounds, with swelling or occasional bleeding, can be the result of endometrial tissue seeding in these sites. And, strangest of all, some women have sought help with nosebleeds which occurred regularly each month, at the same time as their menstrual periods. Again, these were found to be due to endometriosis in the nasal soft tissue.

Vaginal pain around menstruation or during intercourse can be a sign of vaginal endometriosis. So too can bleeding after sex, or having heavy periods.

> About a year after having a hysterectomy for endometriosis, I got out of bed after making love and found I was bleeding. For a few moments, I didn't even recognize anything was wrong. It had always been a joke of ours that whenever I was feeling particularly 'premenstrual' all we had to do was make love and that would bring on my period, and I'd feel better. But, I suddenly realized that I didn't have a womb anymore, so why was I bleeding? We rushed down to the hospital, and they diagnosed bleeding from granulated tissue caused by the operation scars – after the tissue had been stimulated by what they delicately called 'local trauma'. That became our word for it for a few months – 'Fancy a bit of local trauma, then?' However, since I went on to have a recurrence of endometriosis a few years later, I now think that the so-called granular tissue that the hospital doctor had cauterized with silver nitrate, was, in fact, another patch of endometriosis.

How can endometriosis affect you?

Possibly more significant than the symptoms of endometriosis, however, are the *effects* these symptoms could have upon you. By the time they get a diagnosis, women with endometriosis often suffer far more than pain and infertility. Many have had to put up with a mystery and with a degree of humiliation or subtle repression.

I've grown up being apologetic – I'm sorry I have this pain, I'm sorry I'm bothering you, I'm sorry I'm such a bad patient. It extended into my personal life too. I could never scream out that I felt awful or that I wanted some relief and some *help*. I just had to hide my feelings and do my best. Looking back, it all started with our family doctor and a teacher at school. Both of them were so scathing about any complaints of period pains or any slacking.

Pain as a short-lived symptom is unpleasant but can be managed. You grit your teeth until the cause is found and treatment is given, or you swallow pills until the problem goes away. But *chronic* pain – pain which continues or returns regularly – is very hard to cope with. It frays the nerves and makes you tense and irritable. It depresses and tires not only you, but your friends and family who suffer *your* agonies as well. Constant pain baffles and degrades as it saps your energy, your self-confidence and even your self-esteem.

Many women with endometriosis talk in terms of feeling humiliated, let down or rejected during the time between first experiencing the symptoms of the disease and finally getting a diagnosis. Often, the hardest aspect is that the symptoms are so intimate – heavy or painful periods, painful sex or painful urination and defecation – that we can't fully explain them to our friends and family. Or, they are so vague – tiredness, general aches, nausea – that we cannot point to a provable injury. All that can be seen is the result – our apparently unjustified bad temper and our unwillingness to join in with outings or games. Eventually, sympathy gives way to irritation and impatience. The *cause* of all this unhappiness is not seen as the disease – not, that is, until we can point to and *name* a disease – but the sufferer. She becomes the wimp, the spoilsport and the nag.

Pain during sex is particularly humiliating and robs you of the one thing you need when trying to cope with an illness – comfort and closeness.

Depression, however, may be more than just an emotional reaction to what is happening to you. Many years ago, doctors might have talked in terms of psychosomatic diseases, and given the impression that depression was an imaginary disorder. Such a disorder might have been seen as one that did not really exist or had no 'real' cause, and could be cured by just telling the sufferer to buck up. We have now gradually come to understand the strength of the links between the mind and the body.

What is happening in the *mind* – in our thoughts and emotional processes – affects what is happening in the brain, which is the physical and chemical control centre of our bodies. And what happens in the brain affects the endocrine, or hormone, system, and thus the immune system. A lack of self-esteem or a lack of self-confidence can lead to depression. This, in turn, can lead to disorders that make themselves known by purely physical and even measurable symptoms. And the reverse may obviously be true – physical illnesses can, and often do, lead to a sense of failure and misery.

Painful sex can be particularly unpleasant when we are *not* sure why it is happening. The educational and social systems in this country ensure that most of us grow up and enter our first full sexual relationship in utter ignorance of the workings of our bodies. Even if we have learnt about reproduction at school or from our parents, very few of us learn about our sexual feelings or what to expect. We may hear that sex can be physically painful at first, but why this is so is often not made clear. We also often get the impression that men should automatically, and by instinct, know all about sex, how to make love and how to give pleasure to their partners. And that women, to be truly feminine, should be 'innocent', and by that we mean ignorant.

If sex then is painful at first, we assume this is right. If sex goes on being painful, or gradually or suddenly becomes painful, the assumption is often that we are either being punished and deserve this difficulty, or that it is happening because we are somehow making love incorrectly. Very few women will dare to suggest to their partner that he is 'doing it wrong' in case he explodes with fury or asks her how she got to be so 'knowing' that she can say such a thing. Similarly, very few women want to admit that they are deficient in proper female instincts as to not know how to make love painlessly. The truth is, of course, that it takes knowledge and information to understand how our own bodies and those of the opposite sex work. It takes discussion and a sharing of thoughts and opinions to learn how we feel, and how others tick. No one can do this by instinct, and both sexes have equal rights to the facts and the feelings.

Sex, of course, is only one way that you and your partner can show affection and support. And penetrative sex or intercourse is similarly only one way in which you can express your feelings physically. If your condition has led to loving being painful when your partner enters you, try pleasing each other in different ways. It can be just as exciting and even more loving to use your hands, lips and tongues on each other. It can be especially arousing if you enlist the aid of massage or moisturizing cream or oil, to excite and caress each other to satisfaction, without needing to put penis in vagina. We tend to feel that these sort of caresses are childish, because they are the first forms of experiment we enjoyed when we were younger. But if you think of the most erotic film or book you have ever seen to picture really sexy lovemaking, you will realize that actual penetration forms a very small part of the action.

Endometriosis is a hard enough condition to suffer, without all the emotional baggage that might prevent us getting a diagnosis and coping with treatment. Many women may find that to get both a diagnosis and treatment, they need to have more faith in themselves, and need to begin to be a little more selfish. If it hurts, and you know it, *say* so. If you are below par and you *know* something is wrong, *say* so.

The hardest aspect of many endometriosis symptoms, however, is trying to cope with them when we do not know what is causing the difficulties. This is why getting a proper diagnosis (the subject of the next chapter) *is* so very important.

■ CHAPTER FOUR
Diagnosis

I've had various gynaecological problems since I was a teenager. In my twenties, I was hospitalized for PID and continued to get attacks of pain and ill health. I had a laparoscopy when I was twenty-four and was told, quite definitely, by the professor who did the operation that there was nothing wrong with me. So from then onwards, I suffered in silence. I was seen by three different doctors in 24 hours when I had the final acute attack of pain that eventually led to me being diagnosed as having endometriosis. My partner and I were making love and, as he entered me, I felt as if I'd been stabbed with a sword. I work in a birth control clinic, so next day I saw one of the doctors there – a consultant, no less. He suspected an ovarian cyst and arranged by phone for me to be seen by the Senior Casualty Officer at the nearest hospital and to be given an ultrasound.

When I arrived, I was kept waiting for three hours before being seen by a junior doctor who refused to do an ultrasound, refused to let me be seen by anyone else and told me quite definitely that I had kidney stones and they would pass. Next morning, still in pain and *knowing* it wasn't kidney stones, I managed to see another consultant at another hospital. He kept me in for a few days, and then arranged to do a laparoscopy a month or so later. He had a good idea what was the matter, mainly because he listened to me and trusted me. The operation confirmed his diagnosis – severe and extensive endometriosis with cysts and adhesions. I'd spent six years with pain and illness because one doctor had told me there was nothing wrong with me. I wonder how much longer I would have gone on if I had accepted that other doctor's equally certain claim that I had a case of kidney stones?

A diagnosis is important for several reasons, but is not always easy to get – again, for several reasons. The barriers to achieving a diagnosis, what use a diagnosis can be to you and how you can obtain one, are the subjects of this chapter.

If you *do* suspect you might have endometriosis because some of the symptoms described in the last chapter strike an uneasy chord, what would be the point of finding out whether or not you were right? The most immediate and obvious answer is to get treatment. We will look at treatments and their outcomes in the next chapter, but it is necessary to say now that 'curing' endometriosis is not a simple proposition. What *is* clear, is that the longer the disease is left to its own devices, the more damage it does and the more difficult it becomes to remove its effects. A mere six months may be enough to turn a mild case that would respond to comfortable treatment into a serious one that might need invasive surgery or intrusive medical attention, and still leave a legacy of discomfort. This discomfort may not all be physical either, which brings us to the second good reason for getting a diagnosis.

One of the major catastrophes of endometriosis is that it attacks us in our most intimate selves, making private aspects of our lives, such as menstruation, urination, defecation and sex, painful and difficult, and by doing so, it attacks our trust in ourselves. To give them their due, doctors *can* have a hard time diagnosing endometriosis, but to give them due criticism also, many have punished, and still do punish, the women they cannot help.

Doctors are frequently trained to see curing an illness as their only job, and failure to do this as failure on a far deeper level. Doctors often cannot cope with saying 'I don't know what is wrong with you', or 'I can't do anything about your illness'. Some will shift the blame in such a situation by saying, in effect, 'Your disease does not exist. It is all in your neurotic and hysterical mind', or, 'It is all your own fault'. This leaves the patient, already struggling with a burden of embarrassment, pain and confusion, feeling even more humiliated and despairing. Putting a name to what is causing us difficulty and proving that it is *not* the result of trivial hysteria, an inability to accept our own femininity, or our poor sexual relations, can *in itself* help us to feel better.

> After my operation, my doctor told me I had very bad endometriosis. Or, as he put it, 'endometriosis plus, plus, plus'.

> The ridiculous thing is that I felt so relieved. I was vindicated. After years of feeling guilty and being made to feel that my problems were in my mind or that I was lying, I had a *name* to my problem. I had proof that there *was* something wrong. Great!

It is worth remembering in this context that no doctor ever told a man who presented with pain in the groin, penis or testicles, that he felt that way because he could not adjust to his masculinity!

The barriers to diagnosis

You might find three major barriers to getting a diagnosis of endometriosis. Firstly, if you *do* go to a doctor and list one, or a combination, of the main and classic symptoms of the disease, your doctor may not have the knowledge or the experience to recognize the signs, or may believe some of the myths and prejudices that prevent a proper diagnosis being made. Secondly, your symptoms may throw up one or several red herrings; endometriosis can often easily be confused with other conditions. Thirdly, you may be unable to give the doctor sufficient clues or pointers that *could* lead to a diagnosis of endometriosis. You may be too embarrassed to point out that your main or most alarming symptom is painful sex, and only tell your doctor about painful periods. Or you may have been led to feel that pain at these times 'is just a woman's lot', and nothing out of the ordinary to remark on.

> My doctor always makes me feel as if I am wasting his time. I feel stupid and foolish when I talk to him, and I just can't bring myself to tell him any details about my sex life, or about anything else that makes me feel embarrassed. It's just like trying to talk to my father when he's being his most disapproving and hostile. Could you tell your father that sex hurts, when he's sitting there with his mouth screwed up as if everything you say fills him with contempt?

It is important to realize that, when seeking a diagnosis, your first port of call must be your family doctor – a general practitioner. Mark the name well. A GP's skills are *not* those of a specialist. GPs act rather like filters, assessing whether a condition described to them is one that can be dealt with in the surgery or whether it needs further assessment and treatment by a specialist – and if so, *which* specialist. Sadly, some doctors can act, or be seen as likely to act, more like a gatekeepers barring the way than helpful signposts, pointing you in the right direction. Others are only too happy to help, but need *our* full cooperation to be able to do so.

Endometriosis can be enough to baffle the best and most sympathetic of doctors and, of course, if the doctor in the question is *not* the best or most sympathetic, you can have an immediate barrier to getting diagnosis and treatment. As already mentioned, endometriosis is still believed by some doctors to be a disease usually only found in some groups of women. If you do not fall into these categories, you might find your period pains and painful sex ticked off neatly as the result of some other disorder, such as PID. Be aware of this, and be ready to ask about and discuss any diagnosis put forward. Your doctor may have more medical knowledge than you, and should be respected for it. But equally you are more of an expert on your own self, and that should be respected too.

Some doctors still expect the typical endometriosis sufferer to be white, aged thirty to forty, of the middle class, professional, egocentric, underweight and over-anxious. In their view, the classic 'pain in the neck' woman patient! It has emerged, of course, that endometriosis sufferers are not confined to this narrow social, age and racial grouping. The condition *has* been found in teenagers and non-professionals and in married and overweight mothers! It is not then unreasonable, if you are seeing a doctor with symptoms that might suggest endometriosis, for you to raise the subject if the doctor does not.

Conditions often confused with endometriosis

DYSMENORRHOEA

What are the 'differential diagnoses', or the other diseases or problems, you might find a doctor suggesting as the cause of your trouble? For a start, if your main complaint is of painful periods, you may well find your doctor suggests you have dysmenorrhoea. This is not actually a diagnosis, nor is it in itself a disease. It is a description of symptoms. Like so many medical terms, it comes from the Greek, and in this case simply means 'painful monthly flow'. When there is no clear reason for the period pain, it is called primary dysmenorrhoea. The condition becomes known as secondary dysmenorrhoea when the doctor can pinpoint the cause of the trouble.

Painful periods are often seen as a natural part of life and something that comes with the package of being an adult and female. The problem is, of course, that menstruation is surrounded by thousands of years of myth. Men still dominate the medical profession that centuries ago waged a hidden but ruthless war on what were seen to be rivals – the old wise women and midwives who practised a different kind of healing than the medical science, which had its roots in Greece and Rome. One casualty of this war was sympathy or understanding of the *differences* between men and women.

One major difference is that the male body stays essentially static from month to month, and only changes gradually with age. Women, on the other hand, go through a distinct cycle from month to month, as their bodies, and thus their emotions, experience swings and changes. If you set up men as the norm and the standard of what is 'right' and 'correct', then the obvious result is to see women as 'wrong' and therefore, in effect, 'ill men'. The fact that a woman bleeds every month (an act that 'usually' means illness or damage) can be seen by men as profoundly frightening or disturbing.

One way of controlling such fear is to control the woman, and instead of telling her that she has an amazing power in being able to do this, she is told that she is amazingly dirty, or strange or harmful when she does it. And when she complains of difficulties attached to her menstrual cycle, she is told either that it is part of her being a woman ('what can you expect if you insist on doing such a perverse thing?') or that her difficulties are her own fault ('women are supposed to bleed, and if it causes you pain you obviously have a problem accepting your proper sexual role'). Or, there is the suggestion that she is imagining it all – 'show me proof that it hurts, or I'll tell you that it's all in your mind'.

A further cause of difficulties and misunderstanding in all this is that there is no way to *measure* pain. You can measure the amount of menstrual fluid lost during a period, so if your complaint is of heavy periods, this can be shown. But you cannot put a yardstick to pain, and if your doctor is inclined to believe that women are the weaker sex and will make a fuss about nothing, or if you have accepted that pain is something that always happens and must be tolerated, you may find yourself at a dead end.

Periods should *not* be so painful that they regularly disrupt your life and will not respond to treatment. Whatever the age of the sufferer, if pain is not resolved either by an acceptable painkiller or by a short course of treatment such as the Pill, it is reasonable for your doctor to at least consider the possibility of endometriosis. The condition has been found in girls as young as fourteen, so being under twenty is *not* a protection and should not be used by a doctor as an excuse for not looking for this disease.

It has been suggested that women are more likely to develop endometriosis at such an early age if they are born with an abnormality of the genital tract. For instance, an imperforate hymen, where the hymen, or maidenhead (the tag of skin that usually partially blocks off the entrance to the vagina), completely covers the opening. By stopping the exit of menstrual blood until the condition is discovered, this 'outflow' obstruction may encourage endometriosis by increasing the rate of retrograde menstruation. Most girls under seventeen who have endometriosis diagnosed, have suffered from such a problem. Girls with such abnormalities tend to have their difficulties investigated fully. However, when there is no such obvious cause present, girls with dysmenorrhoea can be fobbed off with pills and the reassurance that 'it will get better as you get older, especially if you have a baby'.

MITTELSCHMERZ

Endometriosis may also be misdiagnosed as Mittelschmerz, or 'middle pain', if pain spasms occur at ovulation. Mittelschmerz is a pain that affects some women at ovulation, but, of course, the actual reason *why* ovulation may be painful to you may be because your ovaries have endometriotic lesions or adhesions on them.

SEXUAL AND RELATIONSHIP PROBLEMS

Similarly, painful sex can be dismissed as being a symptom of your having sexual problems rather than being due to a physical cause. It is undeniable that by the time many women see their doctors to complain of finding sex difficult or painful, their relationships are under strain. Stress can lead to increased hormone production encouraging veins in the pelvis to swell and become congested. This causes pain, especially during intercourse. But again this may well be a *result* not a *cause* of the problem.

> I'd already bust up two relationships because of the pain by the time I met Rob. Which meant that *this* time I was really cautious about having sex, and it took ages to get to bed together. So when it *still* hurt, I was devastated. It was Rob who persuaded me that it couldn't be something to do with us or with my sexual attitudes. He said it had to be something medical. He made me see my doctor, and he came with me to give me support. This time, I stuck to my guns and wouldn't accept any suggestion of it being sexual problems. I wasn't going to let this relationship go, and I was right.

PELVIC INFLAMMATORY DISEASE

Endometriosis is also often confused with PID, or pelvic inflammatory disease, and a proper diagnosis is delayed as well-meaning doctors prescribe antibiotics for 'inflammations' that actually need a completely different treatment. If the woman concerned has a sexual and medical history that supports the theory that PID may be the cause of her discomfort, her doctor may not think to look further for the source of her problems, even when treatment does not lift her difficulties.

PID can lead to painful sex, constant nagging discomfort, and to menorrhagia, or heavy periods. All these symptoms could also be present if you have fibroids – bundles of tissue growing within the muscular walls of the uterus. These stretch the area covered by the endometrial lining and cause heavier and painful periods. Kidney stones, similarly, can cause intermittent pain that may be sharp or give a constant dull ache. Sudden onset of a pain located vaguely in the stomach area or radiating up to the collar bone may be suspected to mean an ectopic pregnancy – a pregnancy established in the Fallopian tubes. When this happens, the growing embryo soon becomes too large for the tube, bursting it and producing quite dramatic bleeding and damage.

URINARY TRACT INFECTION AND IRRITABLE BOWEL SYNDROME

Painful urination could be mistaken for urinary tract infection, and painful bowel movements for irritable bowel syndrome. This is another somewhat mysterious condition leading to pain on passing waste matter, diarrhoea or constipation, wind and swelling. A classic sign of it is the passing of mucus from the back passage. It is thought to be a 'stress-induced' disease, that is, a condition giving rise to very real physical symptoms that is caused by emotional upset. It is not unreasonable to suggest that endometriosis and irritable bowel syndrome can be found side by side because the stress of having one gives rise to the other. So, a justified diagnosis of irritable bowel syndrome may not rule out your having endometriosis *as well*!

SUMMARY

In the main, symptoms of endometriosis *can* be distinguished by one cardinal fact. This is that they come and go in time with your menstrual cycle. If your pain, diarrhoea or constipation worsens just before a period and then decreases and disappears only to reappear again a few weeks later, then endometriosis must be suspected. And if menstrual problems do not have another explanation or fail to respond to treatment, always think of endometriosis as a possible cause.

The difficulty is, of course, that having *thought* of endometriosis, you need to have it diagnosed. The very fact that so many of the symptoms coincide with those of other illnesses makes it difficult for a doctor to be sure by just checking off the symptoms themselves. The doctor may not have the full picture, and you may find it hard to lay out every piece of the jigsaw for him or her so that this full picture can be put together. Some women are too embarrassed to say that painful sex is their most noticeable or distressing symptom. Others may not realize that their diarrhoea or tiredness is relevant, or that they are accepting a degree of pain as normal when it is, in fact, a significant pointer to their condition.

Getting a diagnosis

The first step to take on the path to getting a diagnosis, if endometriosis is your problem, is to have confidence when you see a doctor. You must have the confidence to trust yourself and, if *you* think what is happening to your body is troublesome, to say so and stick to your guns. If your doctor says, 'That's nothing to worry about. You have to expect pain/bleeding/loose bowels at your age/after what you've been doing . . .' and you don't agree, then say so. You can always ask for a second opinion if you are not satisfied with what your doctor has done or said. Under the rules of the National Health Service, your doctor does not have to comply if he or she has made a proper diagnosis and nothing more can be done. If, however, your doctor has been unable to do so, or you can persuade him or her that you have good reason to seek further reassurance, you should be sent on.

Doctors have three main options open to them in trying to reach a diagnosis.

MEDICAL HISTORY

A doctor taking a medical history will ask you questions about what is bothering you now, whether it happened before, and how your symptoms have developed. If puzzled by your illness, a doctor may look at what illnesses have affected you in the past and even at what illnesses run in your family. If you have had several sexually transmitted diseases, for instance, this may predispose a doctor to blame pelvic pain on PID. Similarly, a woman with a fat medical file and a history of vague complaints about period pain may find herself stereotyped as 'neurotic' or 'hysterical' – or have an alert doctor suddenly wonder whether endometriosis has been her real trouble all along.

PHYSICAL EXAMINATION

A second option would be a physical examination. Pelvic endometriosis may be 'palpable', or capable of being felt. Adhesions may fix the uterus in place and adenomas might make it feel bulky and tender. A doctor doing a bi-manual examination may feel the raised nodules of endometriotic tissue, or the masses of adhesions along the ligaments, on the ovaries or in the pouch of Douglas. Examination is best done just before or during a period and, again, midway between periods. In this way, doctors can feel the difference. Just doing an examination at midstage can lead to deposits being missed.

Examination can be painful and, sadly, some doctors may be angry or baffled rather than understanding and sympathetic. A doctor may well tell you to relax and imply that any pain on examination is a result of your being tense and not allowing him or her to get on with the job, rather than a valuable clue to what is troubling you.

> He just snapped, 'For God's sake woman, relax' and I burst into tears and said it was nothing to do with relaxing, it *hurt*. He sent

me to a specialist, and it was only when I saw her that I found out that he had written in the referral letter that I had a sexual problem that made me tense up. She was wonderful. She persuaded me to let her examine me, and she was kind and careful. It still hurt, and *she* said that was not a sexual problem, but a physical one. I was then seen by a gynaecologist, and endometriosis was diagnosed. Oh, and I changed doctors!

HOSPITAL TESTS

The final diagnostic tool in a doctor's armoury is a range of hospital tests.

Ultrasound

At present, a doctor might suggest your having an ultrasound. This test involves bouncing sound waves off you, like a radar, with the results building up a picture on a screen that can then be interpreted by a skilled operator. Ultrasound can produce an image that shows if there are unusual masses on the ovaries, uterus or Fallopian tubes. It could sometimes also enable your doctor to see if there are changes to your pelvic appearance throughout the month by doing several ultrasounds a week or so apart. However, even the best operator cannot always tell whether such a mass is endometriotic deposits, a tumour, a cyst or anything else. So, while not being a full diagnosis for endometriosis, ultrasound can sometimes give clues as where to look more closely.

Blood tests

As already mentioned, there is at present no easy or infallible test for endometriosis. There is one under study however that, if successful, could save a lot of money and pain in the future. This is a blood test or, as it is properly called, a serum immunoassay. Studies have suggested that women with endometriosis have a raised level of a substance called CA-125 in their blood, produced by the endometriotic tissue. The reason for this is not clear, but if a test that was highly sensitive to CA-125 could be developed, it might be used to test simply and positively for the presence of the disease.

Immunoscintography

There is also a suggestion that endometriosis might be diagnosed by a process called immunoscintography. In this, a substance that is attracted to CA-125 is injected into the body. If endometriosis is present, this substance will collect around the endometriotic deposits. Since it has been irradiated, it will show up under a special imaging machine. Immunoscintography seems to be successful so far in detecting ovarian endometriosis without the need for surgery. What is now needed is more research and, if this is successful, more money for the equipment to be made available in all hospital gynaecological departments.

Getting a referral for surgery

The only sure way at present of diagnosing endometriosis is by an operation. In the UK, there are only two routes to obtaining this. The first, and in some cases the easier, is impractical for most people. This is to go privately to get an appointment with a gynaecologist, and pay for a diagnostic laparoscopy. If all else fails and you can either raise the money or have it paid for by health insurance, this is an option.

However, the best choice is to go through your own doctor. Many women who are eventually found to have endometriosis have had unpleasant symptoms for some time before finally having the condition diagnosed correctly. This means that if endometriosis *is* your problem, you may have quite a history of interactions with doctors, and they may not all have been pleasant. There is no doubt that most people who go into this difficult profession do so with the wish to help. But there is also no doubt that medical training as it is at the moment encourages doctors to believe in their own authority and infallibility, and to have feelings of anger or failure if they cannot come up with the goods.

Not all doctors are able to say outright, 'Well Mrs Jones, I'm sure your pain is real and has a cause, but I'm damned if I can understand it. I think you should be seen by someone else.' A more common response is likely to be, 'Well Mrs Jones, I think your pain is psychosomatic. After all, you did say you and your husband had not been getting on.' Your doctor may, furthermore, look at your medical notes with despair and think, 'If nothing has been found by *now*, what *is* there to find?'

So, you need to approach the consultation with care and appreciation, whether it is your first or yet one more request for help in a long line of such attempts. Anyone with a professional skill is likely to have their nose put out of joint by the suggestion that a lay person knows more than they do. So going in, waving a book and saying, 'Look here doctor, I think I know what I've got,' is just asking for trouble! But most doctors nowadays support and appreciate the modern trend for people having a better knowledge about their own bodies, and most will acknowledge that patients *are* the best experts when it comes to assessing whether all is well in themselves.

The trick, then, is in both asking for and offering help. You need to go into your doctor's with a very clear idea of *what* is bothering you, and why. The best way to do this is to write down all the symptoms that have troubled you, even the most intimate and embarrassing ones, and explain every one before you leave. If you are going to blush and stammer over some, or feel awkward with too great a list and be tempted to leave some out, write the list out clearly and hand it over for the *doctor* to read.

Have another list of all the questions you want to ask and of all the fears and worries you have. Don't skimp, and don't give in to that dreadful feeling that you are wasting the doctor's time. Remember that this time is paid for out of your and your family's National Health contributions, and your medical treatment is not something offered to you out of charity. It is a service for which you pay, and to which you are entitled. In return for his or her salary, your doctor undertakes to give you all appropriate medical services, and this means proper diagnosis and treatment as required. In fact, the chances are that your doctor will welcome your organized approach.

> I felt an absolute idiot, sitting there with what was almost a
> shopping list and ticking everything off, and I could have sworn
> my doctor had this sort of numb look. I could just hear him
> thinking, 'When is this stupid woman going to finish?' Then at
> the end, do you know what he said? He said, 'Well, Mrs
> Whitehead, you've given me a really clear idea of what is wrong
> with you. I think we can get to the bottom of this now, and I only
> wish more patients would have your sense.' I felt a mile high!

If your doctor is not sure of what is causing your problems, or
does know and realizes that specialist help is necessary, you will
be sent or referred to a specialist in a hospital. If your doctor
does not offer to do this, but either doesn't give you an explanation for your problems or gives you one that you feel is unsatisfactory, you can ask to be referred. The doctor is not *bound*
to give you what you want, but neither are *you* bound to stay in
his or her care. Anyone can change doctors without giving a
reason, and you can do so to find yourself a more helpful one.

The specialist you are most likely to see is a gynaecologist. The
same rules apply here as with your GP. Try to explain everything
that has been bothering you and use notes if needed to give a full
picture. Don't feel intimidated if you don't know the medical
terms, just explain your problems in your own words as clearly as
possible. If this means you have to use 'slang' or 'dirty' words, do
so – it won't be the first time the specialist has heard them! And
if you do not understand anything the specialist says to you, ask
for an explanation in standard English. Medical terms are only
short, quick and precise ways of explaining conditions or appear-
ances, and there isn't a single one that cannot be translated into
simple, everyday terms. It shows a lack in your doctor if he or she
won't do this for you, *not* a lack in you for not understanding.

SURGERY TO DIAGNOSE ENDOMETRIOSIS

Looking for endometriosis is not as simple as it sounds. As has
already been mentioned, the pelvis is not a big hollow cave with a
few clearly marked organs floating in its centre! The pelvis is
jam-packed with organs and fluid and it is extremely difficult to

see exactly what is what. Obviously, if a woman has chocolate cysts or a mass of adhesions and the operation to 'look see' is done just before or during her period, the chances are that the doctor *will* have a clear view of what is wrong. But if the disease has not advanced to the stage of leaving a trail of adhesions, if these and any deposits are small and hidden, or if the operation is done at a time of the month when any lesions are at their smallest, then even a good and conscientious surgeon may miss them.

As we have already seen, the pain and discomfort you may feel from endometriotic lesions are not necessarily in proportion to their size or even their siting. So a doctor can go into such an operation with few or confusing clues as to what is causing the problem. This, in itself, can influence the outcome. The accuracy of any operation to diagnose endometriosis not only depends on the doctor's skills and on the extent of the disease, but also on whether or not the doctor suspects endometriosis, and is looking for it. It was noted in one study that such operations correctly spotted ovarian endometriosis in about seven out of ten cases. But when the diagnosis *before* the operation was of possible endometriosis, the surgeon found it in nine out of ten cases. When the surgeon was looking for ovarian cancer, inflammation in the Fallopian tubes, or an ectopic pregnancy as an explanation for the patient's problems, endometriotic lesions were only found in 50 per cent of cases where they were actually present. These sort of results underline the importance of either you or your doctor raising the possibility of endometriosis if a laparoscopy is to be done in an attempt to find out why your symptoms have arisen.

Diagnostic laparoscopy

What exactly is involved in a laparoscopy? The operation is usually done under general anaesthetic although it is possible, in some exceptional cases, to do it under a local anaesthetic. This would happen, for instance, if there were some good reasons for a patient not being able to withstand the shock of a general anaesthetic. Again, in some exceptional cases, it might be possible for a diagnostic laparoscopy to be done as a day-care procedure, where you go into hospital in the morning and are allowed home that night. On the whole, most hospitals will ask you to come in for an overnight or two-night stay.

As with any operation involving a general anaesthetic, you will be asked not to eat or drink anything for twelve hours before the operation. Do respect this. It isn't a foolish rule to save the hospital money on feeding you! If you have anything in your stomach while under the deep, relaxed unconsciousness of a general anaesthetic, you could vomit. You could then choke to death, or inhale material that leads to infection and pneumonia. Either way, you could kill yourself or give yourself brain damage – or put yourself and the hospital staff to considerable pain and effort. So why risk it?

A laparoscopy is a way of letting a surgeon have a good look at the inside of your pelvis without having to cut you open to any great extent. It is an operation that has only been made possible by advances in medical instruments and training. The tools involved are complicated, and do need to be used by someone who is both skilled and *experienced* for any sense to be made of what may be found.

For the operation, you will be laid on an operating table that tips you up with your feet higher than your head. This position allows the coils of your bowel to slide or be pushed gently up your body and away from the uterus and other pelvic organs. The uterus is usually manoeuvred by the surgeon's assistant during the operation. This is achieved by gently turning an instrument that has been passed up through the vagina.

The surgeon will make two holes in your abdominal wall – one usually near or in the navel, and another lower down. Carbon dioxide gas will then be pumped into you to gently inflate the cavity and allow the organs inside you to ease out and separate from each other. The surgeon uses the higher hole to pass through an endoscope, or laparoscope. These are both names for an instrument like a telescope which, having been passed through your abdominal wall, gives the surgeon a good view inside. The laparoscope, or endoscope, has light passed down it, so the surgeon can see what is going on.

The lower hole is used to pass in other instruments, to cut away adhesions and give the surgeon an unrestricted view, or to push aside and turn your pelvic organs. Fluid will be aspirated or sucked out through this lower hole. The pelvic or peritoneal fluid can then be tested for the presence of antibodies to aid diagnosis. If it contains blood at a time other than menstruation, that can aid diagnosis too. Sometimes, the lower hole is also used to pass a second scope to give a clearer view from several angles.

After the operation, the tiny incisions are closed up with stitches or clips that look like staples. The stitches used may be of the type that dissolve on their own. If not, they or the clips may be removed in a few weeks after the operation by the surgeon or your own GP.

If endometriosis is present, the surgeon may be able to see one or several of the signs of it. There may be blood in the peritoneal fluid. There may be patches of brownish discoloration on the peritoneum, or of blood just under the surface. There may be raised nodules or lumps of a reddish colour, bluish lumps below the surface or whitish nodules.

There may be cysts which can range in size and be reddish or brown in colour. Cysts on the ovary might range from being small and thin-walled, with a noticeably brown or black thick liquid interior, to being large and thick-walled, with a yellow, white or colourless liquid filling. There may be scar tissue around the uterus, ovaries, Fallopian tubes and the ligaments that hold these organs in place, as well as scarring around the bowel and bladder.

If your surgeon does find endometriosis, there are several courses that can be taken, and these will be discussed in the next chapter on treatment. But surgeons will certainly start by making a note on the spot of exactly what has been found during the operation, and possibly even taking photographs or a video film for later study. These records may also be used for comparison. For example, if your doctor considers that you have an extremely mild case, it may be suggested that you wait six months or so to see if treatment is needed. Or, the doctor may wish to put you on treatment and 'look see' six months later to assess if this treatment *is* working.

Classification of endometriosis

There is a drawback here. There are several classification schemes to describe the extent of endometriosis. You may wake up after your operation to be told you have 'moderate', 'severe', 'Stage 1C' or 'Stage II A1' endometriosis. Each term describes the same state, but uses a different classification to do so. The main difficulty with the classification schemes is that they are all developed by doctors looking at endometriosis as an inhibitor of fertility. The lesions or adhesions that lead to a 'high' score and that incline towards a diagnosis of 'severe' are the ones that prevent pregnancy. These, of course, are not necessarily the deposits that cause pain or difficulty.

It is likely that in the future new schemes will be developed to rank pain and the risk of recurrences as well as the possibility of infertility in classifying cases of endometriosis. At the moment, the scheme used by most surgeons is the one drawn up by a panel of experts called together by the American Fertility Society in 1978 and revised by them in 1985. Using this classification, a surgeon looks for lesions, nodules and cysts, and scores points for each one found in specific areas, and for their size. Adhesions are also counted on a rising scale, depending on whether they are 'filmy', light, dense, or extensive.

A woman who has had no discomfort but is being investigated for infertility, may be surprised to learn she has 'severe' endometriosis. On the other hand, a woman who has spent years having pain, difficulties with sex, passing water and moving her bowel may be shocked to be told she only has a mild case. The surgeon is only working with the tools available – in this case, descriptive ones – and is not passing judgement in this assessment. But the sufferer may feel understandably humiliated and rejected to have what she knows is an extreme difficulty dismissed as

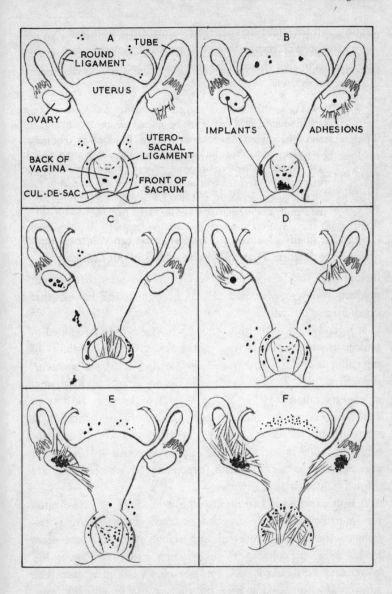

The American fertility chart classification scheme: *(a) Stage I: minimal; (b) Stage II: mild; (c) Stage III: moderate; (d) Stage II: moderate; (e) Stage IV: severe; (f) Stage IV: severe.*

'mild', and therefore 'trivial'. The woman may also fear that her own doctor will respond to this apparent downplaying of her problem, and that this will be reflected in any treatment offered. Of this, more later.

> I was quite shattered and angry when the hospital doctor told me he had found a mild case when he opened me up. I said, 'If that's mild, I hope I never have to get it badly.' But then he went out of his way to explain that he knew that it really didn't mean what it said – mild endometriosis could be even more painful in one person than a severe case in another. He promised me that he took my case just as seriously, and that I would get proper treatment – and I really can't complain about the care I had.

Having finally obtained a diagnosis, what can you then expect from your doctors? That will be the subject of our next chapter.

CHAPTER FIVE

Treatment

> I think the greatest problem you have to overcome as an endometriosis sufferer is *expecting* too much. I mean, most of my generation have grown up with the idea of miracle drugs, miracle cures and miracle operations. If somebody dies in hospital these days, we all want to sue someone, as if dying can't happen unless somebody made mistakes or didn't try hard enough. It's really difficult being told, as my doctor honestly told me, 'I'm sorry, we don't yet know enough about this to make any promises.' I found that my own treatment went better when I stopped feeling angry that it didn't make an instant and complete improvement in how I felt.

Without a 'chemical marker' – a way of using blood tests to tell how far endometriosis has progressed – diagnosis will always be difficult. As we have already seen, surgery is the only way to be sure that endometriosis *is* your problem, and even then it may not give the correct and full picture. The disease is far from simple and the same goes for its diagnosis, so what gave you the idea that curing it would be any easier?

Deciding on which type of treatment to try often depends on the severity of the disease and on how far it has developed. A doctor will also have to consider your age and whether or not you will want to have children in the future. For instance, a woman with extreme symptoms may find that the only effective treatment would be radical surgery removing not only her womb but also the ovaries. Since the ovaries are the main site in the body for the production of oestrogen, and since it is oestrogen that stimulates the growth of endometriotic tissue, if the ovaries cease to produce this hormone, the condition resolves. On the other hand, such a drastic step would hardly suit another woman who is found early on to have a mild case, with some lesions but no adhesions, and is planning to have children. She may find that a course of tablets, followed by a pregnancy, banishes *her* symptoms for ever. Similarly, a woman with the early signs of the menopause may choose to wait out her discomfort since, after the change of life, *very* few women continue to suffer from endometriosis.

Further complications are added by the fact that all the available treatments affect different women in different ways. Some treatments work well on some women yet prove useless on others. Some women also react to a few of the treatments with side effects that can be as unpleasant as the disease itself.

Endometriosis is found to return in as many as one in two treated cases. However, untreated endometriosis, even when not actually giving a problem at the time of discovery, can develop and worsen at an alarming rate. Some treatment is always better than none, and the only real question is *what* treatment and why. It *is* your body, and although your medical advisers might understand the condition and the available therapies better than you can, you still have the right (and, indeed, the responsibility) to learn as much as possible and take an active part in deciding what is to be done. In the end, it should be your decision whether to go ahead with a treatment plan, and whether to continue with it or change it. The more you know, the better equipped you will be to make such choices.

> The doctor went over all the available treatments with me, and it just made my head spin. I said, 'You just give me the tablets and I'll take them. I don't want to know the gory details.' But he said no, I had to understand and take part. He said that I had a better chance of getting well if I wasn't just following what he said. I think he was right. I felt a lot worse for the first few months or so on the tablets, and if I hadn't understood that this was going to happen, and why, I might have just thrown them down the loo. I kept on, and they worked in the end.

Treatment is sought, offered and accepted for two basic reasons – to cure the disease, or to tackle the symptoms. That is, you and your doctor may want your endometriosis to be cured even though it is not causing difficulties, because either or both of you believe that in spite of it not being a problem now, it might be troublesome later. Or, you might demand help from a doctor with stopping the pain without caring whether this involves clearing you of the disease or not. Treatments that cover these intentions fall into the three categories of surgical, conventional medical and alternative.

Surgical treatments

Surgery is essential for diagnosis, and it may also be essential as a treatment. Depending on the extent of the disease, a surgeon may suggest that treatment needs to be 'conservative' or 'definitive'. Conservative surgery is when the patches of endometriotic tissue, cysts and adhesions are removed. Your uterus and ovaries and any affected organs are left intact, and you will still be able to continue to try for a pregnancy. You will not enter the menopause at that stage but may, of course, run the risk of having symptoms return. Definitive surgery means that you will no longer be able to become pregnant as your womb, Fallopian tubes and, most importantly, your ovaries are taken out. The possibility of a recurrence of symptoms is also entirely removed, but you will become menopausal, with all the problems that this might entail.

CONSERVATIVE SURGERY

Some surgeons will take the opportunity, at the same time as making a diagnosis, to remove all the deposits of endometriotic tissue they can find. The limitations of just using surgery to remove endometriotic deposits are twofold. First, even the best surgeon may miss some lesions if they are well hidden or in their early stages at the time of the operation. Secondly, removing lesions active at the time of surgery does not prevent more from appearing later – whether seeded from more retrograde menstruation or from whatever other mechanism that causes endometriosis. Surgery *is*, however, the only way to remove the results of endometriosis, the scar tissue and adhesions that often cause more

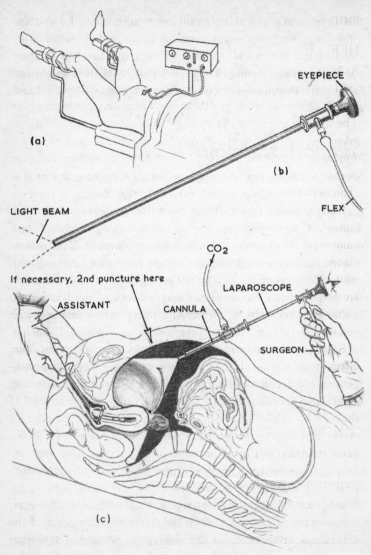

A laparoscope and its use: *(a) introducing carbon dioxide into the lower abdomen, (b) laparoscope, and (c) laparoscopy*

pain and ill health than the endometriotic lesions themselves. Medical treatment, as we shall discuss, can attack the endometriotic deposits, but it cannot do anything about adhesions.

DEFINITIVE SURGERY

As well as cutting away lesions and adhesions, surgery is often used to remove damaged organs if they are not necessary to the body's well-being or if the damage is so extensive as to demand it. The appendix, the uterus and the Fallopian tubes *can* well be taken away with no ill effects – unless in the case of the last two, you want to become pregnant. More important, removal of the ovaries might be the only way you are finally going to be rid of endometriosis.

Endometriosis, remember, is basically triggered off and maintained by the production of oestrogen in your ovaries. Small amounts of oestrogen are created by other means. The adrenal glands produce a hormone that can be converted into oestrogen while being stored in fat deposits in the body, but the amounts are almost always too small to deliver enough of the hormone to encourage endometriotic deposits, which is why the menopause will usually cure endometriosis.

Removing the ovaries before the menopause will have the same effect, since without the ovaries' regular manufacturing of oestrogen, endometriotic deposits will starve and die. For this reason, hysterectomy and bi-lateral oophorectomy (that is, the removal of the womb and both ovaries) are often the suggested treatment for severe and distressing endometriosis. An artificial early menopause can bring other problems.

Artificial menopause

The menopause is, strictly speaking, the last period. However, the stopping of periods is only *one* aspect of what is called the climacteric, or change, and the whole process can take up to ten years to go through its various stages. From the beginning of the climacteric, the ovaries gradually produce less oestrogen until, about half-way through, periods become erratic and finally stop altogether. Hormone levels fluctuate and establish a new and diminished level. In some women, the climacteric is uncomfortable, with the rapidly swinging hormone levels giving rise to unwelcome symptoms such as hot flushes, headaches, insomnia, mood changes and vaginal dryness. In others, the changeover is smooth, with few or no ill effects. A sudden artificial menopause because of a bi-lateral oophorectomy (the removal of both ovaries) is more likely to plunge you into unpleasant sensations.

One of the most dangerous side effects of the menopause, moreover, is osteoporosis. This condition is another reaction to a lack of oestrogen and it happens when calcium is leached from the bones, leaving them lighter in mass, brittle, and vulnerable to damage. The longer you live without producing oestrogen and, therefore, the earlier you enter the menopause, the more bone mass you will lose. This loss can lead to fractures and ill health later in life. So, delaying having the menopause is not just a matter of vanity and remaining young-looking as long as possible, it could be a way of extending your healthy life for a reasonable length of time.

Endometriosis and HRT

So what are your options if losing your ovaries appears to be the *only* way you are going to get rid of your endometriosis? When ovaries have to be removed for other reasons, such as cancer, or when the menopause begins particularly early or brings unpleasant symptoms, most doctors will now prescribe HRT – Hormone Replacement Therapy. Oestrogen or, in cases where the woman concerned does still have her womb, oestrogen and progestogen, are given on a regular basis. The artificial hormones fend off all the unpleasant symptoms that the menopause can bring, including osteoporosis. HRT can be taken as a tablet, inserted as an implant or, more recently and very successfully, passed into the body through a skin patch – a see-through sticking plaster that is replaced twice a week.

The $64,000 question is, of course, whether these doses of artificial oestrogen will act in the same way as your own natural oestrogen and restart the endometriosis. There have been cases reported of this happening, although they do not appear to be common. Since all symptoms do resolve in such a situation as soon as the HRT is discontinued, it would seem to be worth trying, as long as you *do* see your doctor if the trouble starts again.

Medical opinion appears to be divided on how long women can, or should, continue taking HRT. Some doctors suggest a year or so, just to tide you over the period during which your body adjusts to a lower, and then minimal, level of oestrogen. Others say longer. Obviously, a woman entering the menopause artificially at a young age because of the removal of her ovaries may be advised to go on taking hormones until the age at which she would have been expected to enter the natural menopause. What is clear is that taking HRT, even for a few years, extends a protective effect against osteoporosis for some time afterwards.

LASER SURGERY

Endometriotic deposits are usually removed by being cut out, or they are cauterized or burnt with an electric current (diathermy). The difficulty is, of course, that any damage to tissue from either technique *could* lead to further scarring, and the development of either adhesions or of a perfect site for new endometriotic tissue. Furthermore, the heat produced by diathermy can be enough to damage tissue lying next to the operation site. The bowel and the ureters (the tubes that pass urine from the kidneys to the bladder) are particularly at risk of being damaged in this way.

A new technique uses a laser to burn tissue. This has been found to be far less dangerous and seems to be more effective than other methods. This is because the surgeon has far more precise control over the depth that a laser burns, and the heat produced is confined to a smaller area. A laser also vaporizes the abnormal tissue and adhesions as it cuts them out, reducing the risks of scar tissue *resulting* from the very operation that seeks to eliminate it. Lasers are, however, still fairly rare and very expensive, and special expertise is needed to use them, so they are unlikely to be available to the majority of women currently going for treatment. This is a pity since their use gives a further advantage. Diagnosis and the removal of deposits from mild endometriosis are likely to be done via laparoscopic or endoscopic operations. These, as described in the previous chapter, are not intrusive operations in that they do not require a long hospital stay or a large incision in the body.

If the surgeon finds extensive endometriosis, however, and needs to cut and remove considerable areas, a bigger operation is likely to be scheduled. This is a laparotomy, when an incision is made just below the bikini line. The scar will probably only be a few inches long, but it will be larger than the tiny holes needed for a laparoscopy. Laser therapy, even to remove quite extensive endometriotic areas, can be done endoscopically.

SURGERY FOR PAIN

One further treatment that can be given surgically is for certain nerve pathways to be cut so that the message of 'pain' is not transmitted from its site to the brain. Pain may originate in your little toe, forefinger or right ovary, but unless the fact travels up through the necessary nerves to the brain, it doesn't actually register there and bother you. In cases where nothing else stops the discomfort, pain can be relieved by blocking these pathways, without ill effects.

Conventional medical treatments

Endometriosis relies on chemicals involved in your menstrual cycle to trigger and enlarge its development. There are three stages in a woman's life when endometriosis does not seem to develop – before she starts her periods, when her periods are in abeyance due to pregnancy, and after her periods have finally stopped. All, to be precise, times at which she is not ovulating and not producing any significant amount of oestrogen, or is also producing a high level of progesterone at the same time. And, of course, *men* do not develop endometriosis unless they too are subjected to a high level of *female* hormones. Most medical treatments to get rid of endometriosis itself are variations on duplicating three of these states artificially: being post-menopausal; being pregnant; and being a man.

There are drawbacks involved in each therapy, as will be discussed, and there is one drawback overall. This is that endometriosis and its treatment have no certainties. The traditional advice has been to get pregnant, the assumption being that in the nine months of high progesterone production, the endometriotic lesions will wither. However, there have been reports of women who have emerged from a pregnancy with a baby *and* a continuing case of endometriosis. In some women, having a pregnancy does work, but in others the lesions may increase in the first three months, decrease for the next six months and then resume after the baby is born. There have also been a few cases of women whose bodies still manufactured enough oestrogen after the menopause to sustain their endometriosis. No case has yet been reported of a girl with endometriosis before her periods have started, but that may be because we have not yet found one, not because none exists.

So, even if each medical treatment did what it was intended to do, and put you artificially into a pregnant or menopausal state, this may still not produce the desired result. In addition, we are not dealing with bacteria that can be killed, but with tissue that grows in response to a delicate balance of hormones and other body chemicals. Getting the balance right, to undo harm without causing more, is tricky. So, what medical treatments are available?

DANAZOL

This is the most popular drug used to treat endometriosis. Popular, that is, among doctors but not necessarily among patients. Danazol works by putting your body into a more masculine state. Prescribed under its trade name of Danol, danazol is a derivative of a synthetic form of the hormone testosterone. Testosterone is one of the hormones we call 'androgens', that have a masculinizing effect, just as oestrogen has a feminizing effect. It is the hormone responsible for the development of male 'secondary characteristics', such as heavy muscles, body hair and a deep voice. Both men and women produce a small quantity of these 'gender' hormones of their opposite sex. Men have some oestrogen in their make up, and women some androgen.

Danazol has several effects on the body which can make it extremely effective in dealing with endometriosis. Firstly, it has an anti-gonadotrophin effect. That is, it interferes with the pituitary's production of the gonadotrophins FSH and LH in the menstrual cycle (see Chapter 1). Because the surge of these hormones is reduced, endometrial tissue in the lining of the womb and endometriotic tissue in any lesions do not receive the full message to thicken and grow. Danazol also directly affects the ovaries and these are not stimulated, as they would be normally, to produce oestrogen. Thirdly, danazol increases the amount of testosterone circulating in the system. The result of this is an 'anti-oestrogenic' state – one in which oestrogen production is discouraged and oestrogen is largely absent from the body. Without active oestrogen, most endometriotic deposits shrink and die away.

It is worth noting, however, that danazol can only help to resolve the actual patches of endometriotic tissue. Scar tissue or adhesions are unaffected. This means that danazol has been found to be a very effective treatment on its own in mild or moderate endometriosis and in cases where, for instance, period pain was the main complaint. When endometriosis is severe, that is when adhesions have become a major part of the problem and when chronic or all-month-long pain is the trouble, or when large ovarian endometriomas are involved, danazol may only be useful as *part* of the therapy.

Danazol can be offered in doses of 200 to 800 mg daily, and should be taken two to four times a day as each dose wears off fairly quickly. It does need to be taken over four to six months for it to have a proper chance to work. The problem with the drug is that, in some women, it can have some fairly unpleasant and even long-lasting side effects. These can be severe enough to make it very difficult for you to last out the necessary treatment time.

> Within a few weeks of starting danazol, I came out in itchy bumps
> all over my legs, body and arms. It didn't seem too worrying, just
> a bit noticeable. My doctor said he had never heard of this being a
> danazol side effect, but that I should stop taking it. As soon as I
> did, the bumps went down.

During danazol use, your body is losing feminizing hormones
and having a higher level of masculinizing ones. You may find
that your facial and body hair thickens and increases while your
head hair can become thinner, your skin becomes spotty and your
breasts shrink. Some women have reported voice changes, with a
deepening of tone and loss of control similar to that found in
teenage boys when the voice 'breaks'. Depression, tiredness,
muscle cramps, joint pains and hot flushes have all been reported
as other side effects.

> I've had painful knee joints ever since I took danazol, even though
> I was only on it for a few weeks the first time, and for around two
> months on the second course. It's now some three years ago, and
> I still ache every morning when I get up, and I have to be careful
> if I jump over fences or anything when we go walking, because
> that can hurt.

> It's very difficult to describe what happened to me while taking
> danazol. I got depressed, but it wasn't just that. I lost the ability
> to concentrate, so that I couldn't sit down and do any work.
> Thoughts and ideas slipped through, like sand through your
> fingers. This continued even after I'd stopped taking the tablets.
> In fact, I lost about six months. I would have failed my degree if
> it hadn't been for my doctor, who was really good, and my tutor
> who spent hours giving me extra tutorials when I finally got back
> to normal.

Some doctors suggest that regular exercise can help with the
undesirable side of danazol treatment, and it has certainly been
proved that a good work-out three times a week can make an
enormous and beneficial difference to your mood, your health
and your weight. The only drawback with this is that, thanks to
those male hormones, you may still gain weight when doing
exercise. It will not be fat, however, but muscle bulk. In effect,
you will be undergoing a drug and training regime similar to the

one that some athletes follow secretly, and get banned from their sports for doing if they are caught! You may still retain this gain when you have finished the danazol therapy. The good news, however, is that women have different profiles to men, and instead of building up bulging lumps on their arms and shoulders, women develop a firm outline which can be far more attractive than the usual 'flab'!

Your periods are likely to stop during danazol therapy, although this is not essential for the treatment to be effective. What *is* essential is for you not to become pregnant during the therapy, as danazol can be passed to a baby through the placenta and may cause cancer or masculinize a female foetus. Danazol is considered to be an effective contraceptive in itself, but you may feel safer using a condom or cap just to make sure. Since you will be taking danazol to block oestrogen production you cannot stay on the Pill, if this is your form of birth control, while you are using it. Some women find their sexual appetite decreases with danazol use, but others have reported the rather startling side effect of an increase in size of the clitoris and a heightening of sexual urges.

> The funniest side effect was that I felt randy virtually all the time I was on the damn stuff. My clitoris sort of tingled constantly. But it actually wasn't very pleasant because, instead of feeling sexy, I just felt jumpy and a bit resentful. It went away as soon as I stopped the treatment.

Most of these side effects go away as soon as danazol therapy is finished. A few may remain, and this is why it is important to evaluate and discuss them as they arise and to consider if they justify stopping the treatment. Voice changes, for instance, can be permanent, as can pains in the joints. Danazol can also have a lasting effect on the blood that could make you more prone to heart attacks later on, and it can affect blood sugar levels, the thyroid and the liver. For this reason, it is unwise to take the drug for longer than six months at a time.

GnRH (LHRH) ANALOGUES

Concern over the side effects of danazol and the need to find another therapy for women not helped by it have led to a search for alternative ways of causing 'medical oophorectomy' – chemical methods of stopping the production of oestrogen from the ovaries. In other words, duplicating the post-menopausal state. The removal of the ovaries is, of course, the best way of doing this, but risks of osteoporosis or a desire for the woman to still keep the possibility of having a pregnancy mean that a temporary and reversible menopause would be a better option.

A range of synthetic substances has been developed that act on the pituitary. These are gonadotrophin-releasing hormone (GnRH), also called luteinizing-hormone-releasing hormone (LHRH) analogues. This means they are substances that act like the chemicals that tell your pituitary to produce the hormones that trigger oestrogen production.

GnRH analogues can be either agonists or antagonists. An antagonist inhibits the release of hormones, and would work by discouraging the pituitary from producing its hormones. An agonist works by initially stimulating the pituitary, giving it a kick so that it produces hormones full time instead of in pulses as it normally would. The result of this is that the pituitary switches off or 'down regulates' and slows down its production of LH and FSH. After the initial 'kick', the levels of these gonadotrophins drop fairly quickly and in three to six weeks, oestrogen levels will be low enough for endometriosis tissue to be affected.

GnRH agonists can be given in three ways. As goserelin (trade name Zoladex), it is implanted in a slow-release capsule placed under the skin which lasts for four to six weeks. Buserelin (trade name Superfact) is a nasal spray, and naferelin is taken orally two to three times a day.

The GnRH analogues have a similar range of side effects to danazol, although the androgenic, or masculinizing, effects are not so marked. They more resemble those that can be experienced in the menopause. There can be hot flushes, dryness in the vagina, night sweats, insomnia, vaginal 'spotting', loss of sexual feelings, tiredness, irritability, depression, joint stiffness and tender breasts. However, studies comparing the two treatments seem to show that GnRH analogues produce less weight gain, less water retention and less depression, but more hot flushes. GnRH analogues do not appear to have the same undesirable effects on the blood that danazol can have, but they do seem to encourage the shedding of calcium from the bones. This shedding can lead to osteoporosis, and has led to some researchers suggesting that calcium supplements should be given along with this therapy. Bone mass will be made up after the treatment ends, but, as with danazol, this does put an approximate six-month time limit on the therapy before there is a risk of the cure being worse than the disease.

GnRH analogues do seem to clear up endometriosis and to reduce some pain. But, as with danazol, these drugs act only on the endometriosis itself, not on the resultant adhesions. Another minus is that symptoms may get *worse* for a short time after treatment begins, before they get better.

THE CONTRACEPTIVE PILL

As has already been explained, endometriosis thrives in a particular hormonal state, when the woman's body is receiving a regular and continuous oestrogen stimulation. It is more than likely that the lifestyle of women in the last quarter of this century has been encouraging to this disease. Unlike our great-grandmothers, we do not spend a large part of our lives being pregnant or breastfeeding. Instead, having had our first period at around the age of twelve, we then continue to bleed and ovulate every month, with perhaps nine, eighteen or, in a few cases, twenty-seven months out, for the next thirty-five to forty years. Even if we take the combined oral contraceptive Pill, we use it in such a way as to encourage a regular, if lesser, period of bleeding each month.

The advice to have a baby to 'cure' endometriosis is based on some truth. Frequent pregnancies can be discouraging to the disease, and the time off to produce a child *can* relieve the symptoms. However, it may not be the hormonal state of the nine months of pregnancy that has this effect. The first three months of pregnancy may actually *increase* the symptoms and the growth of endometriotic deposits. It is the last part of the pregnancy and the first few months of motherhood, *if you breastfeed* that can possibly create the correct state which effects a cure or resolves some of the lesions – a state of anovulation, when ovulation is not happening and oestrogen is not being manufactured by your ovaries.

We have looked at how drugs can help by changing your hormonal state to one more like a man's, or to one more like that of a menopausal woman. Drugs can also be used to attack endometriosis by mimicking pregnancy. This is done by taking a combination of oestrogen and progestogen – in other words, the combined oral contraceptive Pill. The difference, however, is that for the therapy to work, the Pill must be taken continuously. This means taking it *every day*, instead of the usual contraceptive usage of taking it for twenty-one days followed by a seven-day Pill-free break.

At first, the lining of the womb and any endometriomas will 'decidualize', that is, grow and thicken. But as therapy continues, the tissue atrophies or withers. The natural processes of the body take care of this dying tissue. Combined-Pill therapy does seem to be effective, but less so than danazol. However, if you have been on the Pill and find it suits you, and other drug therapies do give rise to unpleasant symptoms, this may be worth trying. Pill therapy is usually offered for a period of six to eighteen months.

The combined Pill can, of course, have its own side effects such as weight gain, nausea, depression, headaches, loss of sexual feeling, and breast tenderness or enlargement. More important, your blood pressure may rise, and the risks of developing a clot in a vein – thrombo-embolism – can increase. When this therapy was first used, before the advent of danazol or GnRH analogues, the dosage was fairly high. Contemporary contraceptive Pills contain a lower dose, and a medium-dose Pill would seem to be just as effective, while lessening the possibility of side effects.

Pills used so far have been combinations of lynoestrenol and ethinyloestradiol (trade name Minilyn) and norgestrel and ethinyloestradiol (trade names Trinordiol and Logynon). New combinations, such as ethinyloestradiol and desogestrel or Gestodene (trade names Mercilon, Marvelon, Femodene and Minulet) are supposed to have less harmful effects on blood profile, but have not yet been studied fully in the context of treating endometriosis. They may turn out to be an effective and less risky alternative to the pills in current use.

It is the oestrogen in the combined Pill that increases your risk of getting harmful side effects. Because of this, many doctors who are trying to offer the Pill as an alternative to danazol now suggest using a progestogen-only Pill. This therapy still mimicks the pregnant state, when progesterone levels are high and, just as with combined-Pill therapy, makes endometriotic tissue grow at first and then die back.

Treatment is usually for six to nine months, but can be for longer. Therapy can be in tablet form – norethisterone (trade name Primolut N) or dydrogesterone (trade name Duphaston) – or as an injection using medroxyprogesterone acetate (trade name Depo-Provera) which is given every three months. Side effects can be break-through bleeding, weight gain and fluid retention, breast tenderness, nausea and depression. Some users have described the effect as being much the same as having a continuous bout of premenstrual syndrome. If you *are* unlucky enough to react to progestogen and suffer any of these side effects, you can stop the treatment at once if you are using pills. But if you have had the injection, you are stuck with them until the injection wears off.

GESTRINONE

Gestrinone is a relatively new drug – a chemical of the same group that makes up the sex hormones – which has effects similar to danazol. It appears to block oestrogen from endometriotic tissue, encouraging it to break down, and also appears to discourage the ovaries from producing hormones. Gestrinone seems to relieve pain well, and clears up lesions.

Its side effects can be the same as with danazol – oily skin and acne, increased body hair, head hair loss, breast reduction, nausea, constipation, bloating, muscle cramps, hot flushes, voice change, increased sexual urges and increased clitoris size. It is taken by tablet two to three times a week for six to eight months, or can be given as an implant that lasts a year.

TAMOXIFEN

Tamoxifen (trade name Tamofen) is a drug that suppresses oestrogen. It is usually used in cases of breast cancer where the tumour responds to this hormone. It also seems to suppress the growth of endometriotic tissue. In a very limited study, it appeared to give relief from endometriotic pain and to resolve endometriotic deposits in women who had not been helped by other therapies. Reported side effects have included hot flushes, constipation, acne and tiredness, but these stopped at, or soon after, the end of treatment.

PROSTAGLANDIN INHIBITORS

Prostaglandins are chemicals made by body tissue, and have various roles. They regulate menstrual bleeding by passing the message to the tiny muscles and veins in the uterine wall to start sloughing off the lining of the womb, and then to close again. They also tell the walls of the uterus to contract during menstruation and during childbirth, to force out the contents of the womb.

Prostaglandins are also a part of the body's natural healing and defence system and are manufactured by the body as a response to any injury that causes inflammation and pain. They act directly on pain receptors and sensitize them. Women with endometriosis do seem to have higher than normal prostaglandin levels, and it would seem that these substances are produced by endometriotic tissue. The more endometriotic tissue you have, the more prostaglandins you may have circulating in the fluid of your pelvic cavity. For this reason, drugs that block the action of the prostaglandins may help, at least, with any pain caused by the condition and be more effective than other pain-killers such as aspirin or even codeine. Drugs such as mefenamic acid (trade name

Ponstan), ibuprofen (trade names Apsifen, Brufen), or naproxen sodium (trade names Naprosyn, Synflex and Laraflex), specifically block prostaglandins.

Alternative or complementary treatments

Many endometriosis sufferers have turned to alternative medicine either because conventional therapy has let them down, or because of what they see as the need for some sort of control over their own bodies and their illness.

HERBAL MEDICINE

Many of the herbal remedies are, in fact, just a different and possibly less alienating form of the drugs we buy from a pharmacist and that are made in a laboratory. It is worth remembering in this context that a chemical is chemical, whether we call it a 'drug' or a 'natural remedy', and whether it comes from a multinational drugs company or as part of a tea packed by your local health shop. However, proponents of herbal medicines point out that a specific substance which has not been isolated, but is offered in such a way that it is buffered by other components, has a gentler effect on the system. Many herbal remedies, such as Echinacea, or Purple Coneflower, work by strengthening the immune system, and so stimulating the body's own defences.

Evening Primrose oil

Evening Primrose oil has been suggested as helpful to endometriosis sufferers. This is hardly surprising, since it contains a substance called gamma-linolenic acid (GLA) which can encourage the body's ability to synthesize one particular type of prostaglandin, and so help with pain and inflammation. The oil is available from most chemists or health-food shops, under the name of Efamol. The suggested dose is two or three 500 mg capsules, twice a day after food. Other sources of GLA are safflower oil, borage-seed oil and blackcurrant-seed oil.

Evening Primrose oil is most often used in the treatment of premenstrual syndrome and fibrocystic breast disease. It has been noticed that better results with these problems are obtained when the oil is supplemented with vitamin B6, vitamin C, zinc and magnesium. Niacin has also been suggested as a supplement. For this reason, Efamite – which contains vitamins B6 and C, niacin and zinc sulphate – is offered for use in conjunction with Efamol. The same may be true when Efamol is used for endometriosis.

SELENIUM

Another nutritional addition that has been suggested is the trace element selenium. This seems to strengthen the immune system and to have an anti-inflammatory effect. It is obtainable as Selenium ACE, a preparation that includes vitamins A, C and E, all of which help the effect, and is taken as capsules once or twice a day. You should note here that to make the preparation easily processed by your body, selenium is cultured with yeast. If you are someone who suffers thrush, this may bring on an attack. So, ask your chemist or health store for an inorganic or yeast-free form of selenium.

VITAMIN E

Vitamin E is another substance that has a role in affecting the body's immune response. It modulates the synthesis of prostaglandins, and an endometriosis sufferer may find that extra vitamin E helps with pain. The vitamin is also said to prevent scar tissue from thickening. However, it has also been suggested that since vitamin E *deficiency* leads to infertility in rats, it might have an effect on oestrogen in the body. It could then activate endometriotic lesions on the one hand while helping symptoms on the other.

DIET

Vitamins, minerals and trace elements can, of course, be obtained from your diet. In many cases, this can be done just as efficiently, and a lot more cheaply, than buying them in pill form. A healthy diet would benefit you in every other way as well, so it might be worth your while making a real effort to overhaul your eating habits.

GLA is present in cold-pressed safflower oil, which can be used to cook with or in salad dressings. Green, leafy vegetables give you magnesium, vitamin B (if it is cabbage), and vitamins C and E. Nuts and seeds will increase the amount of zinc, magnesium and niacin you eat, and offal will give you niacin, magnesium and vitamin B6. Oily fish, such as herring or tuna, will bump up your intake of zinc, niacin and selenium.

In fact, if you want to look good and feel good, you should throw out all your convenience foods, cut down on animal fats and sugar (that means fewer fried foods, biscuits and cakes) and make sure you eat plenty of wholewheat cereals, breads and pasta. Eat plenty of fresh fruit, salad and vegetables, and more fish, lean meat, nuts, seeds and beans.

If you want extra vitamin B6, concentrate on wholegrains and wheatgerm, have plenty of offal, such as liver, and eat red meat, black molasses, eggs and cabbage. If you feel you need vitamin C, stock up on fresh fruit, particularly citrus fruit, and fresh vegetables, especially of the leafy green kind, such as spring greens, spinach and lettuce, and tomatoes. Remember to have these raw or very under-cooked since vitamin C is destroyed by cooking. If you want vitamin E as well as vitamin C, enjoy avocado pears with your spinach – both are good sources of these two vitamins. Other sources of vitamin E are eggs and oily fish such as herring, tuna (fresh or tinned), fresh sardine and mackerel. These are also a good source of zinc. Vitamin E is also found in good quantities in vegetable oils, nuts and wholewheat cereals.

Sources of GLA are blackcurrant-seed and borage-seed oils, and cold-pressed safflower oil. All these can be found in herbal or health-food shops. If you want extra niacin in your diet, eat plenty of fish of any type, red meat and offal, wholegrains, yeast, peanuts and beans. The body can also process niacin from eggs and milk. Magnesium is present in some fruit such as apples, grapefruits and dried figs, and in some leafy green vegetables. Cereals, other vegetables, red meat and offal are other good sources. Selenium is found in broccoli, garlic, onions, tomatoes, tuna, wheatgerm and wheatgerm oil. Zinc is available in most nuts, molasses, oysters, seeds such as sunflower seeds, wheatgerm and wheatgerm oil.

Pain-killers

As well as using anti-prostaglandin mefenamic acid (Ponstan), there are various ways of killing endometriosis-induced pain. You may find you need additional help to enable you to cope with pain while other therapies are attacking the endometriosis at source. Or, you may have taken the decision not to use another therapy at all, but just to deal with this particular symptom.

Several methods harness the body's ability to manufacture its own pain-killing substances. These are called endorphins, and are chemicals made in the brain that relieve pain in the same way that morphine or other opiate drugs would do – but naturally, and without the same addictive effect. Endorphins are derived from an amino-acid found in the brain and also in the pituitary gland. Amino-acids are the building blocks of protein. Endorphins are usually broken down fairly quickly by the body, so one way of getting pain relief is to take a natural amino-acid which inhibits the enzymes that would otherwise break down the pain-killing endorphins. DL – phenylalanine (DLPA) – appears to do this, especially if taken with vitamins B6 and C. It may take a few days for the therapy to work but the effect then lasts for some time and can continue even after the pills have been stopped.

ACUPUNCTURE

Endorphins can also be stimulated by means of acupuncture. In this therapy, sterile needles are inserted in specific points on the body. They only penetrate a few millimetres and, after being twisted gently, or even having an electric current passed down them, they are left for a short time. The usual explanation of their effect is that the needles are put in at some point along the fifty-nine meridians, or energy pathways, that cover the body, and that this encourages the body's natural energy to flow and heal. A more modern, and probable, explanation is that the therapy encourages the body to produce endorphins, with a very beneficial result.

> I was amazed to be offered acupuncture by the physiotherapist at my Health Centre. I thought it was a fringe medicine and couldn't be found on the NHS. I was also sceptical about its effects, but I had to eat my words. It really does work, and it helped me tremendously.

EXERCISE

Another way of getting your endorphins going is by taking vigorous exercise every day. A proper work-out – one that raises your pulse considerably and holds it at an elevated level for at least 20 minutes, getting you hot and sweaty – will make you feel relaxed, more energetic and less in pain. If you are unhappy at the idea of using surgical or medical ways of removing or switching off your ovaries, you might consider Nature's way of doing it. You will also do wonders for your figure, if you have the time for this amount of physical activity. In fact, serious and vigorous exercise will deal with endometriosis by putting your body into the first state during which this condition does not arise, that of a pre-pubescent girl. Athletes such as marathon runners, who undergo extensive training that severely reduces the amount of fat they carry, frequently find their periods stop, their breasts become smaller and their body hair decreases.

> I do a work-out every day, either on my way to work or on the way home. I used to say I never had time for any keep-fit, but in fact that's just making excuses. You can fit it in, and I wouldn't do without it now. I have a really bad case of endometriosis that won't respond to treatment. But as long as I don't miss my exercise classes, I feel fine and stay OK.

TENS

Yet another form of pain relief is TENS (transcutaneous electrical nerve stimulation). This works on the principle that the pain messages travelling to your brain can be blocked or confused by a tiny electrical current which 'short circuits' them. You are given a small battery-driven device that is connected to two electrodes. Every day, you stick these to your skin near the painful area, and switch the device on. You then turn up the voltage until you just feel a slight tingle and leave the electrodes in place for an hour or so. This can be surprisingly effective as a pain reliever. Some women find it only works while the device is on, or for a few hours afterwards, but others report a whole-day benefit. TENS can be especially helpful in dealing with chronic or lasting pain, and for women who do not want to take drugs continuously.

Pregnancy

Pregnancy has, quite seriously, been suggested as a cure for endometriosis. It is true that many cases of primary dysmenorrhoea do clear up after a pregnancy, and that many endometriosis sufferers have improved after giving birth. But this approach has similar drawbacks to most of the other therapies. That is, it is uncertain, there is no way of telling before trying it out whether it will work at all, or how well, and the side effect in this case is a very long-term one. It means sixteen to twenty-one years of full-time dependency and a lifetime of responsibility! Surely, children are too important and too precious to be conceived purely as a measure to rid yourself of a disease?

> I've had my family, so it really got on my nerves the way I kept being told that the best way to cure endometriosis was to have another baby. It didn't cure me last time, so why should it now? And it seemed such an intrusion – being told to have a baby, but not for the baby's sake.

Of course, if having a child is what you and your partner have planned and wanted, then a possible resolution of your endometriosis would be a happy extra. But, even then, you might find that it is not conclusive. However, it does seem that many women, while finding their endometriosis gets worse in the first trimester of pregnancy, do then improve. Extending the period of anovulation – the time during which you don't ovulate – increases your chances of this working, so it will help if you breastfeed for as long and as frequently as possible after the birth. Breastfeeding or lactation, when done 'on demand' and little and often, keeps your body in an anti-oestrogenic state.

Summary

In practice, very few endometriosis sufferers will try one and only one of these treatments. To be most effective, many of them need to be used in tandem. Surgery, for instance, is often best after a course of danazol or GnRH, when all but the worst of the lesions may have shrunk, and the surgeon's job is then mostly to remove adhesions. Diet, exercise and non-prescription remedies often aid prescription drugs, as well as helping you to feel more in control of what is happening to you.

The drawback of *all* the treatments we have reviewed, apart from the removal of the ovaries, is that there is no guarantee that the whole process will not start up again and endometriosis return. There is no way of telling, either before or after treatment, whether you are going to be one of the lucky ones, experience a complete resolution of lesions and not have a recurrence, or whether small deposits will remain and grumble on to put you right back at the beginning again in a few months or years. Even the severity of your symptoms is no guide. Serious cases have cleared and remained clear, while mild states have proved difficult to eradicate.

If endometriosis *is* your problem, you might have to prepare yourself for a psychological battle as much as a physical one. While it is obviously unfair and trivializing to *dismiss* the endometriosis sufferer as having a condition that is 'all in the mind', we do need to understand and accept the influence our attitude can have on our physical well-being.

A lot of research is now going on in a new field of medicine called psychoneuro-immunology. This is looking at the very complex interactions between the brain, the hormone system and the immune system. We know that our emotions can have a very significant effect on the workings of the hypothalamus. This, in its turn, switches the pituitary on and off. The pituitary drives the whole hormone system, and this system can have a very significant effect on the body's defence mechanism against ill health.

You may take for granted the fact that being ill will lead to your feeling miserable. But we can now go one step further and say that when you experience an emotional 'low', body chemicals circulate that physically slow you down. What begins as a feeling in your mind becomes an actual bodily state, which is why it can be hard to pull yourself out of this situation. Illness may also create these mood chemicals, so that the emotional state is manufactured in the body along with the other chemicals that serve to inflame tissue and make it sensitive.

What is important here is that the reverse is true. A lot of complementary or alternative medicine treatments harness the mind's powers over the body. They are based on a belief that if you approach a therapy with determined optimism, you can drive all your mental and physical mechanisms towards well-being, rather than towards ill health. It is obviously dismissive and foolish to simply tell someone who is feeling awful to 'pull their socks up', but it has been shown that the more you programme yourself towards being well rather than ill, the better your chances are of defeating any disease.

Your attitude can affect you in other ways, too. It is easy, after many years of undiagnosed endometriosis, to become a victim. If you have always had your pain and discomfort subtly put down as imaginary, and your efforts to find an answer described as 'neurotic' or 'hysterical', you can emerge feeling crushed, querulous, of low self-esteem, slightly guilty and hard done by. A consequence of this may be that you get into the habit of making the most of your misfortune. For example, when you don't feel well, vigorous or happy enough to go bounding out in front of the group, enjoying life and having fun you may *use* your illness to force your friends and family to hang back with you.

If you are to tackle your endometriosis, either to cure it or at least to cope with it, you first need to see how you might be using your illness to your advantage, and how you might actually be better off letting go of it. It might seem strange and even insulting to all those women who have had so much pain, to suggest that they may be benefiting from their discomfort, but we do need to face our innermost fears and needs when it comes to chronic illness, and make sure that one part of us is not sabotaging our expressed wish to find a cure.

Many people find it is particularly helpful to get in touch with other endometriosis sufferers, and we are lucky in Britain to have a well-organized network of self-help groups which have been set up by the Endometriosis Society. It can, at first, be depressing and frightening to share experiences with other people and to find out just how many women have suffered terribly from endometriosis. But there can be no doubt that self-help groups are enormously supportive, and it can be such a relief just to know that you are not alone and that you have been neither over-reacting nor imagining things. Other sufferers at different stages of the disease can give you the confidence to persist, or be examples of when to call a halt on an unproductive treatment route. The Endometriosis Society also has the support and encouragement of leading researchers in this field, and can keep you up to date on the latest developments.

CHAPTER SIX

Endometriosis and Infertility

> I want a baby, desperately. I've always wanted children. I come from a big family and, somehow, having lots of children has always seemed the natural way to me. I can't accept that we are a *real* family until we can have a baby.

Getting pregnant is a bit like looking for a policeman – never there when you want one, and always arriving when you don't! It's a sad truism among gynaecologists that their work seems to split evenly between helping teenagers who desperately don't want a pregnancy, and 'fell' first time, and mature women who desperately *do* and can't seem to find the switch after trying for ten years. What is often forgotten is that pregnancy is actually a delicate balancing act to achieve. For a baby to start, a whole chain of events must click into place at the right time, and both your and your partner's bodies do have to be in optimum condition. Even a small change in your hormones or other body chemicals, and you will not succeed. So to understand how endometriosis and infertility might go together, you must first remind yourself of how a pregnancy *is* started.

Getting pregnant

The male contribution is sperm, and this is manufactured continuously in the man's testicles. Sperm is pushed out from the testes via two tubes called the vas deferens. These meet in the prostate gland, where sperm and seminal fluid are combined to make semen. At ejaculation, up to 300 million sperm will be present in the teaspoon or so of fluid that emerges – 98 per cent of which is the protective seminal fluid. Having been deposited at the neck of the womb, the sperm will try to swim up the uterus and to the top of the Fallopian tubes.

The first barrier it encounters may be a physical one. Mucus at the neck of the womb is designed to form a protective plug to keep foreign material out of the uterus. For most of the time, this mucus is thick and opaque. Except, that is, just before ovulation when it becomes clear, thin and stretchy. The mucus actually forms channels, funnelling the sperm up the vagina and through the os. The environment of both vagina and uterus at this time of the month is welcoming to the sperm.

The sperm itself, of course, must be able to make and survive the journey. For the male partner to be fertile, his sperm must be 'motile', or able to move well, and healthy. Even the most welcoming environment cannot hurry on sperm that is slow, sluggish or damaged. However, in some cases, the mucus in the vagina remains hostile at all times, and even healthy sperm may be trapped and unable to survive.

Having travelled through the uterus and Fallopian tubes, sperm must encounter a fertile egg at the right time. For this to happen, the woman's menstrual cycle must proceed (as outlined in the first chapter) until an ovum is released. This ovum is wafted in the fluid that surrounds the pelvic organs and moves towards the open ends of the Fallopian tubes. Tiny hair-like organisms inside the tubes, called cilia, wave rhythmically and set up a current that draws the egg towards the tubes.

The meeting of egg and sperm must take place at the right time. Sperm, we believe, can survive for up to five days, but may be weak and on its way to decaying by then. The egg is only in its best state in the first twenty-four hours of ovulation, after which it begins to decay. Only one sperm will break through the ovum wall and fertilize it, yet evidence shows that many sperm must surround the egg for this to happen. A lone sperm or one in scanty company will not succeed. If egg and sperm meet, and conditions are right, fertilization will take place and the resulting bundle of cells – called a blastocyst – continues its seven-day journey down the Fallopian tubes to the womb. It then implants in the womb lining and continues to develop.

This process can be interrupted in a myriad of ways. Any disturbance in your hormonal system can mean that an egg may not mature, that it may not be released, or that it may be damaged. Sperm may be prevented from travelling up the womb and Fallopian tubes, or damaged on its journey. The egg may not be able to reach the Fallopian tube itself, or may not be able to continue down. Once in the womb, it may fail to implant, or may do so but then soon be shed. Many of these difficulties are to be found in women with endometriosis, and may or may not be directly connected to the disease.

Is there a link between endometriosis and infertility?

There seems to be no doubt that endometriosis and infertility have some sort of connection. Various studies suggest that 25 to 50 per cent of infertile women have endometriosis, and that 30 to 50 per cent of women with endometriosis are infertile. However, we have so far not been able to fully answer the obvious question – does endometriosis cause infertility, or does infertility cause endometriosis? Or, indeed, are both caused together by a third factor?

We do not have exact figures for how many women actually suffer from endometriosis, but it may be far more than is presently estimated. Experience does seem to confirm the view that endometriosis is less common among women who have had children without difficulty than it is among women who have had problems becoming pregnant. However, it may be that a large number of mothers have had endometriosis, or have gone on to develop it, but that, for many reasons, their condition has never been diagnosed.

The available information can be used to argue each theory

about the nature of the link between infertility and endometriosis and this is not just of academic interest. If infertility is caused by endometriosis, and if it is your primary, most distressing symptom, it would seem logical that curing endometriosis should enable you to become fertile again. If, on the other hand, endometriosis is caused by infertility, merely trying to treat the endometriosis itself might not work: you might have to tackle at source the causes of your infertility to have any lasting effects on the disease.

How may infertility cause endometriosis?

As we have already seen, endometriosis may not in itself be a very unusual condition. Looking at any of the theories on how it arises – the implantation theory, the coelomic metaplasia theory, etc. – we can see that the longer the span between a woman starting her periods and her first pregnancy, the longer her body is subjected to a highly oestrogenic state, and the more likely she is to develop endometriotic deposits outside the uterus. By not having a child, her body is denied the protective effects that a lack of ovulation due to pregnancy and breastfeeding would offer.

There are various theories describing how and why endometriosis can render a woman infertile. Some studies seem to indicate that women with endometriosis are likely not to ovulate every month. It has also been suggested, although most studies so far do not support this claim, that they are more likely to suffer luteal-phase defects. These arise when the corpus luteum (the area on the ovary left behind by the matured egg), that *should* trigger the production of progesterone, is deficient. If too little progesterone is produced, or if enough is produced, but for too short a time, a fertilized egg cannot implant in the womb.

A pregnancy can only occur when all the subtle ups and downs of hormone production are in balance. Too much or too little of any of the vital hormones will mean that the system cannot work properly. The hormones produced by the pituitary and the ovaries are obviously important, but so too are the substances, such as adrenalin, testosterone and prostaglandins, that are produced by other sources in the body. It is worth noting, for instance, that many couples are convinced that they can remember the exact lovemaking which led to the conception of a wanted child, and that it was especially pleasurable. Rape victims, on the other hand, have a greater statistical likelihood of falling pregnant from their assault than would be expected. The role of hormones, such as prolactin and adrenalin, whether produced from pleasure, fear or a defect in the body's system, may be surprisingly important here.

Several studies also suggest that endometriosis has as variable an effect on women's fertility as it does on any other symptom. In spite of the fact that most of the classification systems specifically score on parameters that have to do with fertility, one woman with mild endometriosis might have great difficulty in becoming pregnant, and another with a severe case may succeed easily. Similarly, just treating the endometriosis may not result in a pregnancy and a successful outcome might require other treatments as well.

How may endometriosis cause infertility?

The most obvious way in which endometriosis might cause infertility is when cysts or scar tissue actually form a physical barrier to a pregnancy taking place. Scar tissue can prevent the free movement of the pelvic organs. For ovulation to be effective, the fimbria at the ends of the Fallopian tubes need to pull closer to, and hover over, the ovaries as an egg is released. If a major part of the ligaments supporting the ovaries, tubes and uterus is bound up and twisted by adhesions, this movement of the fimbria may not be able to happen. Scar tissue can also loop around the Fallopian tubes, crushing them shut and so preventing the egg travelling to the womb.

Scar tissue, inflammation and endometriotic deposits could also cause infertility in another way. If sex is painful, a couple may avoid lovemaking altogether, or experiment with different positions and techniques that were found to lessen the woman's pain. This would make her more comfortable but could mean that the man does not ejaculate deep inside her, which might then reduce her chances of achieving a pregnancy.

Contributory factors

LUF SYNDROME

Women with endometriosis, and those with an otherwise unexplained infertility, have often been found to suffer from luteinized unruptured follicle syndrome (LUF syndrome). This is when follicles in the ovaries respond to the surge of LH early in the menstrual cycle and start maturing their egg cells, but none actually breaks open and rupture to send out an egg.

LUF syndrome is yet another example of the conditions surrounding endometriosis about which it cannot be said with absolute certainty whether they are a cause or an effect. Women who have been positively identified as having LUF syndrome are also found to have a low concentration of progesterone in the fluid that is found in the peritoneum. Low progesterone favours the implantation and growth of endometrial tissue, so that the woman suffering from LUF syndrome may well go on to develop endometriosis. However, this is still debatable, since no study has proved that *high* levels of progesterone in the peritoneal fluid *prevent* endometrial cells from implanting and developing, although it is suggested that this is an important factor. Additionally, some progesterone is still produced by the cells of these follicles even though none of them has undergone the full change to becoming a corpus luteum.

LUF syndrome can be difficult to diagnose because hormone levels in the woman's body in the second half of her menstrual cycle – sharply rising levels of progesterone and rising levels of oestrogen – still seem to indicate that ovulation has truly taken place. LUF syndrome is arguably only confidently diagnosed if a doctor can *see* via a laparoscope or a skilfully administered ultrasound, that none of the ripened follicles actually has a ruptured wall.

PELVIC INFLAMMATORY DISEASE

It has also been said that women with endometriosis are often found to suffer from salpingitis, or inflammation of the Fallopian tubes. The Fallopian tubes are the site most often infected by pelvic inflammatory disease (PID), which is an inflammation in various organs in the pelvic cavity, triggered by untreated or intractable sexually transmitted disease. PID is one of the most common causes of infertility as it stops pregnancy by creating scar tissue in the Fallopian tubes. PID and LUF syndrome are then both put forward as third factors – conditions that could give rise to *both* endometriosis *and* infertility.

ABNORMAL PROLACTIN PRODUCTION

Some research has further suggested that women with endometriosis have abnormal prolactin production. Prolactin is the hormone that sets off milk production in the breasts. Endometriosis patients are sometimes found to have galactorrhoea, which is when milk can be expressed even if the woman is not, and has not recently been, pregnant. However, there is still not enough evidence to confirm a definite link between excessive prolactin levels and endometriosis.

Autoantibodies

Infertility may arise in women with endometriosis because of a high level of autoantibodies. Remember, one theory is that endometriosis is an auto-immune disease that develops when the immune system is not able to stop the products of retrograde menstruation from implanting in the wrong environment. Antibodies are produced to try to cope with this invasion, and the theory is that they then react against the lining of the womb itself and interfere with the implantation of an embryo, triggering a miscarriage. What is more, these antibodies may also cause the womb to be hostile to sperm as it makes its way up through the uterus towards a rendezvous with a waiting egg.

Endometriosis may cause infertility by further altering the make-up of the peritoneal fluid. Endometriotic tissue in the pelvis sets up inflammation, and this may have many effects. It may increase the number and the activity of the macrophages, the scavenging cells that usually deal with invading particles or damaged cells. Most studies show that women with endometriosis have significantly more macrophages than women without the disease. The macrophages can attack sperm and treat it as if it was invading bacteria, slowing it down or destroying it as it travels through the womb or through the Fallopian tubes.

Prostaglandins

It has also been suggested that changes in the peritoneal fluid interfere with the ability of the fimbria – the hornlike ends of the Fallopian tubes – to pick up the ovum as it leaves the ovary and starts on its journey to, and then down, the Fallopian tube. However, another constituent of peritoneal fluid may have some effect on the fertility of women with endometriosis. As already mentioned, such women have higher levels of prostaglandins – chemicals that, as well as other functions, have an effect on pain response and womb contractions. It is believed that some prostaglandins are involved in making an ovum burst out of a follicle, but if prostaglandin levels are too high, the ovum cannot emerge.

High prostaglandins may also stop the Fallopian tubes from helping an ovum along its way down towards the uterus. A fertilized egg may then take so long to make this journey that the lining of the womb is no longer able to support a pregnancy when the ovum finally arrives. Another theory is that it is prostaglandins that stop the corpus luteum producing sufficient progesterone to prepare the lining of the uterus, causing the luteal-phase defects mentioned earlier on. And last of all, elevated prostaglandins may stimulate the uterus to contract and to cause a very early abortion, or simply discourage the fertilized egg from implanting.

Endometriosis appears to have a direct effect on the ovum itself, and that means that even IVF, or 'test tube', birth may be less likely to be successful for the endometriosis sufferer than for other women with infertility problems. Eggs which have been removed and combined with sperm in the laboratory are half as likely to become fertilized if they come from endometrial women than if they come from women whose infertility has another cause.

Your chances of a pregnancy

It seems that even mild endometriosis reduces your chances of achieving a pregnancy by four to six times. Having suffered endometriosis, even though your Fallopian tubes are unblocked and your ovaries clear, can reduce your chance of becoming pregnant each month by a factor of 20. *But*, there seems to be little evidence that even apparently successful treatments of endometriosis can guarantee a cure for infertility. This is why researchers are still unsure which causes which. Women with infertility problems found to have mild or moderate endometriosis and treated with danazol have gone on to become pregnant. But so have others who took no medication but just kept on trying to get pregnant. Some women whose other symptoms were cleared by danazol have continued to be unable to produce a baby.

There is little research on whether treatment with GnRH analogues, Gestrinone or combined oestrogen and progestogen results in better pregnancy rates. Some studies point to success, but they are either small or uncontrolled. There is certainly no clear *proof* that medication on its own in treating endometriosis will also treat infertility. Neither is there proof that surgery will necessarily do the trick. This is not to say all of these treatments will *not* work, it is just that we do not yet have the clear and unequivocal proof that they *do*.

If infertility and endometriosis are your problems, what you and your partner choose to do must depend on your individual needs and on a joint decision between you and your medical advisers. Sadly, it must be accepted that a surprisingly substantial number of couples – as many as one in six – have problems having a child, and that one in ten of us will have to make the best of an alternative lifestyle to the classic '2 parents and 1.8 children' type of family.

A family *is* still a family when it contains two adults, or two adults and one or more children not related by blood. Although we can point to couples who have finally succeeded in producing their own child after years of treatment, the fact is that the longer you have to continue trying, the less successful you are likely to be. Some clinics and doctors will continue to treat you, keeping up your hopes and allowing you to put as your only criterion of success the eventual production of a baby. Others will ask you to call a halt, and to channel your energies into accepting the situation and establishing a new goal – looking after someone else's child, looking after each other, looking after yourself.

> I do still have a lingering sadness that we couldn't have children of our own. However, I do think that the doctors who tried so hard to help us, kept us back in a way. I wasted several extra years trying for something I wasn't going to get, and it put a blight on our marriage that lasted for some time. In the end, we woke up one morning and realized how lucky we were to have each other. We now have a child of our own. Someone else gave birth to him – and he has a father we don't know – but he's our child none the less, and we love him, and each other.

CHAPTER SEVEN

Questions and Answers

Considering that endometriosis has been known about for 130 years, why can't the medical profession cure it?

Because, in spite of the myths some doctors (and patients) would like you still to believe, the medical profession is *not* all-knowing and all-powerful. We know a staggering amount of information about the human body today and can, compared with the last century, work many medical miracles. But there is infinitely more to be learnt, and infinitely more work to be done. While being awe-struck at the amazing advances we have seen in surgery, chemistry and genetic manipulation in our time, we must not fall into the trap of demanding that doctors *must* know it all, or be held up as failures.

The problem with that attitude is that it causes many members of the medical profession to become defensive. Since they *can't* understand and cure everything, they may feel inadequate if called upon to do so. It is not surprising that some of them then are evasive. In effect, they say, 'No, I'm not a failure, *you* are. Your disease does not exist, and you're making it all up. Or it's your fault, anyway.' By all means push for more research and for more knowledge, but accept that there are still limits at the moment, and that this is no one's fault. There are *still* 'more things in heaven and earth, than are dreamt of' in present-day medical science.

Ever since I was diagnosed as having endometriosis, my husband has been very 'off' with me. I think that he is afraid he might catch something from me if we made love. Is this possible?

No. Endometriosis is not a disease that can be caught from anyone. It is a condition that comes about because of a complex number of reasons that have to do with the workings of your own body. Another woman couldn't 'catch' it from you, no matter how intimate you were with her, and a man most certainly cannot.

I have the feeling that merely reassuring him that he can't be made ill from contact with you would not be enough to banish his fears and confusion. Men have a difficult time when the women they love develop any form of gynaecological disorder. We bring them up in our society to be proud of their strength and power, and to express this forcefulness in their sexuality. The very words we use to describe their sexual parts, feelings and behaviour – a prick, feeling horny, having it off – are couched in hard, damaging terms. It is then small wonder that when their partners are taken ill with some disease or damage to their sexual parts, most men feel a profound and secret guilt. Because they are also brought up to hide and deny their emotions – especially those that make them vulnerable – very few are able to face and discuss their fears. They react by stonewalling, or by trying to shift the blame by attacking their partners before anyone can attack them for causing the problem. If one of your symptoms was painful sex, your husband may well be feeling angry and terrified that someone is going to point the finger at him, the brute, for doing this to you. One way of his avoiding confrontation is to then withdraw. Both of you need to talk about this, and it might help to do so with the aid of a counsellor.

You say that one theory about the origin of endometriosis is that it happens when cells change. This sounds a bit like having cancer. Is endometriosis a form of cancer, or can it become cancer?

Endometriosis is not cancer, but you are right in seeing a link. Cancer itself is not a case of cells going rotten or becoming diseased, but one where cells that have a specialized job suddenly go out of control, multiply and stop performing a specific function. The difference, perhaps, is that cancer cells stop other cells performing and, by definition, are abnormal. Endometrial tissue *has* a function, and by that definition is normal tissue – even if, as endometriotic tissue, it is doing its job in the wrong place! What is abnormal is not the tissue, but the site.

Having said that, it must be admitted that cancer is sometimes found in the same area as endometriosis. What is as yet not certain is whether this is a coincidence, or whether the endometriotic tissue has undergone a malignant transformation to become a form of cancer. It can be depressing enough to have endometriosis without carrying around the fear of its becoming cancer, and statistically it is highly unlikely to do so. However, it is a good argument for having even mild endometriosis treated, rather than leaving it to its own devices.

I have dreadful period pains, and have had them for years – I'm now eighteen. Does this mean I have endometriosis?

Not necessarily. However, even though you are still in your teens, it *is* a possible diagnosis that should not be dismissed. If your doctor has not already considered this as the reason for your problems, do ask for it to be investigated properly. It may certainly be worthwhile asking for a referral to a gynaecologist for a discussion and an examination.

My doctor has been fairly helpful with my endometriosis, except for one thing. I did have PID a few years ago, after catching gonorrhoea, and I get the distinct impression that he thinks my endometriosis is no more than my just deserts. I'm feeling bad enough already with this.

I wonder if he is as judgemental with his bronchitis or lung cancer patients, giving *them* the impression that if they must smoke, what can they expect? It's a sad and strange fact that many people still have special rules when it comes to diseases caught by sexual contact which they don't apply to disease developed as a result of any other contact or act. Measles can be sexually transmitted too, but you don't get the sort of social distaste if you catch that illness that you do if you catch gonorrhoea. Neither do we allow ourselves to be burdened with guilt for having the former, while we do for catching the latter.

Catching gonorrhoea is nasty, bad luck. Yes, you should have taken precautions and used a condom. But, since you can catch an STD as a virgin and on your wedding night from a loving husband who himself has only ever had one other sexual experience, it is hardly relevant to be terribly moralistic about it. You could be just as judgemental with those conscientious idiots who insist on going to work with just a little dose of cold or flu, and pass it on to the whole office!

I hope your doctor *isn't* being judgemental, and that it is actually your own guilt and unease that are making you read disapproval into the situation. The cure for that is for you to realize that notions of blame and fault are simply inappropriate and unproductive here, and to throw them overboard. If you then still feel a slight coldness in his treatment of you, tell your doctor that you think his attitude is unfair, impertinent and far from helpful.

I've been seeing my family doctor, off and on, for years about painful periods and painful sex. He offers me pills, or tells me to see a marriage guidance counsellor. I can't change doctors since we live in the country and the nearest other doctor said we were too far away for him to take us on his list. Are there any other ways I could get help?

If your doctor flatly refuses to send you to a hospital for tests, there are a few strategies that can get you to someone else who will look at these symptoms and try to explain them to you to your satisfaction. There will be a family planning clinic, or a travelling doctor doing family planning sessions, in your area on a regular, if infrequent, basis.

Doctors who do family planning sessions usually interpret their work as covering a range of 'Well Woman' checks, and will almost certainly be happy to see you and talk to you about this problem. Your local hospital *may* also run a 'Well Woman' session or centre, and these are open to any woman and do not require a letter from your own doctor for you to get an appointment. If all else fails, it might even be worth attending the sexually transmitted disease or urino-genitary clinic in your hospital, which will also see you without a referral letter from your doctor. Yes, I know that your problem is not related to such a disease, but actually half the patients seen at such clinics are *not* suffering from an STD.

The ethical situation here is touchy. If a doctor at one of these clinics – excepting, perhaps, at a urino-genitary one – did feel that you needed further tests or a treatment different to that being offered by your own GP, he or she would be bound by the clinic's own rules to contact your doctor and send you back to him for further referral. This could be difficult. In exceptional cases, a clinic might make its own referral and inform your doctor. It really all depends on how the clinic doctor you see feels able to justify the situation.

Another route is to 'go private' and pay for the consultation, either at charitable organizations such as the Marie Stopes clinics, or at one of the private health groups. BUPA and PPP run their own centres offering 'Well Woman' check-ups, as do private establishments such as the Nuffield hospitals, and the Cromwell hospital in London.

The private health sector insists on sending the results of any findings back to your own doctor. The advantage of this is that at least you have a written second opinion that backs up your wish for further, specialized investigation. Your doctor may then react with petulance and anger, or be relieved that someone else has finally unravelled the mystery of your problems.

I seem to spend half my time in my doctor's surgery. I've had period pains as long as I can remember, but I just can't get my doctor to take me seriously. My medical notes are about two inches thick, and I can just see him screwing up his face in annoyance every time I come in. All he does is reach for his prescription pad to give me pain-killers and tranqs. I want neither. I want help, and I want to know what is wrong with me, because I know something is wrong. Any suggestions?

When trust has broken down between a doctor and patient, it is often difficult to rekindle it. It sounds as if your GP has given up trying to look for a physical explanation of your symptoms, and has consigned your case to the realms of emotional upset. However, even if he was right in this diagnosis, he might be more helpful if he offered you counselling rather than pills.

I think the only option in a situation like this is to call it a day and seek a new doctor/client relationship. Under the rules of the National Health Service, you can go to another doctor in your area and ask to be taken on to his or her list, if the doctor of your choice has room. You don't have to tell that surgery or the one you are leaving your reasons for changing. If you are not able to find a surgery that can fit you in, you can go to the governing body of your local GPs – the Family Practitioner Committee – and ask them to find you a place. In that case, of course, you don't have a choice and may be jumping from the frying pan into the fire!

The best way of making a proper choice is to ask among friends and neighbours to find a doctor who *listens* and explains, and who is willing to be a partner in your quest for a healthy lifestyle, rather than The Boss over your illnesses. The main point to remember when approaching a doctor is that medical advice is a service like any other. When you call in an electrician, you expect expertise and you expect service. You obviously bow to the professional's greater knowledge in some things – when your electrician refuses to put a wall plug in the bathroom, this is for a good reason – but you also expect a degree of courtesy and discussion over what you think needs doing, and why.

It may sound heretical, but a doctor is not very different from other professionals. For a start, a doctor's services are not a free, charitable donation. Doctors' salaries are paid out of our NHS contributions and calculated on the basis of how many patients are signed up with each surgery. Your doctor is paid an amount for having you on the list, and is paid additionally for extra treatments you have, such as contraception or immunization.

Doctors are human. Most are deeply caring, aware, and very keen on their patients having a say and responsibility for their own health. Some, however, are impatient, arrogant, unsympathetic and inclined to be judgemental and influenced by prejudices and myths. And even the best doctor can, like the rest of us, have a bad day or get off on the wrong foot with a particular patient and never be able to repair the relationship.

Doctor and patient relationships are two-way. You can't expect the doctor to do his or her best if you aren't also giving full information and being totally honest about your fears and needs. You also owe it to both of you to have confidence in your knowledge of yourself. If your doctor says that something is unimportant and you are sure it is not, SAY SO. This will tell your doctor that either the diagnosis needs to be examined further, because you may be right, or that the way it has been explained needs to be modified because you are not convinced, and need more information and reassurance.

You have certain rights in this relationship. You have a right to be seen by your doctor at any time during surgery hours. The only exception is if your doctor has made it clear that an appointment is needed, in which case you must be given such an appointment within a reasonable time. You have a right to 'reasonable skill and care' in a doctor diagnosing and treating you, although you have no right to say what that treatment should be. That is, you can't demand pills when the doctor does not think them appropriate.

You can refuse an offered treatment. You can ask for a home visit, but your doctor has the final say on whether you should come to the surgery or be seen at home. You can't insist on a 'second opinion', if your doctor feels it isn't necessary. However, a doctor does have a duty to seek one for you if he or she is not sure about what is wrong with you, or about what to do about it. You don't have the right to say which hospital you are sent to, nor who you should see – but, again, you can say if you have a preference and your doctor should at least listen to you.

If you ask for information about your illness, your doctor should answer truthfully and fully. Doctors may want to keep quiet about certain things if they think it will worry you unduly. Nevertheless, you have the right to ask for full information even though, at the moment, you can't insist on seeing your medical notes. This may soon change.

If you have any worries or complaints about your doctor, the best people to ask for advice are the Community Health Council. These are health watchdogs, and every area has a local office which will be listed in your telephone book. There is also an organization, called the Patients Association, that looks after our interests and can be extremely helpful. If you chop and change too often between doctors, you may quickly get a reputation as a 'troublemaker', and be refused a place on a doctor's list. Doctors have a right to choose too! However, if we don't exercise our right to vote with our feet when doctors *don't* make an effort, we discourage the many good ones and encourage the few who are inconsiderate. As in all consumer matters, we owe it to ourselves and everyone else to ask for and to support quality of service.

I caught gonorrhoea when I was a teenager and I didn't go for treatment until I had quite bad pains. I apparently had pelvic inflammatory disease, and I've now been diagnosed as having endometriosis. What is really frightening me is that my doctor might tell my husband about my past.

Your doctor is duty bound to keep any information about you confidential. Obviously, the facts must be passed on to any other medical professionals involved in your case, but they are strictly forbidden to discuss them with anyone else – even your nearest and dearest.

If you haven't shared what happened in your youth with your husband – and I can see that it might cause difficulties – then you might like to tell your doctor that it *is* a part of your life you don't want your husband to find out about. But it certainly shouldn't come out from your doctor, and it need not be revealed by you. Although PID *might* be a condition that predisposes you to developing endometriosis, this is by no means certain, and it definitely isn't the only theory to explain this disease. So, in trying to tell your husband why you have this distressing problem, you don't have to tell him about your past.

I'm on the Pill, and I'm worried in case the extra oestrogen I'm putting into my body makes me more likely to develop endometriosis.

When you take the combined oestrogen/progestogen contraceptive Pill, it is not really a case of *adding* hormones to your body. What is actually happening is that these artificial hormones discourage the pituitary from producing FSH or LH, and so the ovaries from producing oestrogen. Rather than adding, you are substituting!

I'm twenty-five and in good health, but I'm worried that I might develop endometriosis. This isn't a silly fear – both my mother and sister have it. I've also decided that I don't want to have children for quite a few years, and maybe never. Is there anything I can do to reduce the risks? I am on the combined Pill for contraception.

Yes, you can manipulate your Pill usage to put your body into a state less likely to encourage endometriosis. The combined Pill already imitates pregnancy to a certain extent in that it levels off your oestrogen production, eliminating ovulation. However, the original inventors of the Pill decided that women would feel happier having regular bleeds while taking it, to reassure themselves they were not pregnant, and to be more 'natural'. For this reason, you have a Pill-free seven days every three weeks, and during this time the drop in the hormone levels is enough to cause a withdrawal bleed. Oestrogen in the Pill is then enough to allow the endometrium in the womb to grow, before shedding again.

Endometrial tissue *can* establish itself outside the womb under this regimen, even though it will be less prolific than if you were not taking such medication. However, if you take the Pill *continuously*, rather than breaking off every three weeks, the endometriotic tissue will wither. Researchers have suggested that taking the Pill for four to six months at a time and only having periods two or three times a year, would actually be healthier on *all* counts than having periods thirteen times a year.

Considering the fact that our great-grandmothers had later menarches, the menopause earlier and far more pregnancies than we do, you can see that it is far more 'natural' to have fewer periods. If the combined Pill has already been passed as safe for you, the risk of its possible side effects will not be increased by your taking it continually. Furthermore, by doing so you will also protect yourself from some disorders such as anaemia and some cancers. Obviously, ask your own doctor, but it might be a sensible course for you to consider.

I have had endometriosis which has been treated successfully, and recently gave birth to a daughter. One thing worries me, will I pass it on to her?

Endometriosis does not seem to be a hereditary disease in the same way as is, say, Huntington's Chorea, where children of an affected parent have a fifty-fifty chance of also developing the disease. Nevertheless, sisters and daughters of endometriosis sufferers *do* develop the condition at a slightly higher rate than the unaffected population – which, more than just coincidence, may indicate that there is some inherited common factor.

However, you should not feel guilt, or fear that you have doomed your child to having problems. What you might like to do, though, is to pass on the benefits of your experience. If, as a teenager, she does have painful periods, be perhaps a bit more aware that endometriosis may be a possibility than most parents and doctors usually are in this situation. And when she gets to an age when contraception is a sensible subject, be positive about the benefits of the combined contraceptive Pill. Suggest that she uses this, not only as a birth control, but as a way of cutting down on the number of bleeds her body experiences before she has children. If she decides to opt for a child-free lifestyle, ask her to seriously consider continuing use of the combined Pill for its protective effect against possible endometriosis.

We've been trying for a baby for four years, and ten months ago I was diagnosed as having endometriosis. Yet, miracles of miracles, I've now discovered I'm three months pregnant. I'm overjoyed at the thought of having a baby, and I'm also wondering if this will cure my endometriosis. Will it?

It might, especially if you consider a few simple actions that will be helpful on all counts. If you haven't already decided to breast-feed, think about it now. Breastfeeding is best for your baby, since it not only allows both of you maximum closeness, but it also passes on valuable protection against childhood illnesses. Most important for you, breastfeeding will hold your body in a hormonal state that is hostile to endometriosis.

In the first three months of pregnancy, you will probably still have enough oestrogen circulating to allow endometriotic deposits to go on growing. The last six months will be 'anti-oestrogenic', and those patches of endometriotic tissue will have begun to wither, die away and be absorbed by your body. The longer you can go before your ovaries get back to normal and produce oestrogen, the better. If you breastfeed 'on demand' – little and often – your body will hold off. It does mean you will be tied, since the effect is dependent on *constant* stimulation. If you try to take short cuts to get yourself some rest – such as expressing milk so that your partner can bottle-feed the baby in the night – you may well allow ovulation to begin again.

Breastfeeding will be tiring and time-consuming, but it may well be worth it. By the time your baby is ready to take solid foods and feed to a routine, you should have given your body ample time to clear the endometriotic deposits you had.

I'm having treatment for endometriosis, but I'm getting very uncomfortable side effects. Should I stop taking the medication, or keep plugging on?

You should see your doctor as soon as possible and discuss things. Some side effects produced by some therapies do create real problems, and these can become permanent if allowed to continue. Others, although distressing, are not dangerous and will go away as soon as you stop the treatment. It might be worthwhile gritting your teeth for a month or so of discomfort in order to complete a course and succeed in dealing with the underlying disease. But you do need to talk to your doctor, to determine which category your difficulty comes into, before you make any decision.

My doctor wants me to take a six-month course of tablets for my endometriosis. I've heard that these drugs can have some side effects. Is this true?

We have found that some of the medication that deals best with endometriosis can sometimes have side effects which may be permanent. Women who have taken danazol have experienced voice changes – a deepening and a weakness in tone – that remain even after therapy has finished. Other sufferers have complained of joint pains that came on during this treatment and did not go away afterwards.

To have some effect on the disease, some therapies *do* have to produce major changes in your body, and we can't always be sure that they will pass completely. The only thing we can do is to ask you to weigh up the pros and cons of drug therapy, alternative therapy and no therapy. If you do decide that your symptoms make it wise to try some form of orthodox medical treatment, keep in close contact with your doctor and monitor what is happening in your body. Any changes should be discussed, and if you *are* reacting in a way that you find intolerable, or that experience suggests could leave permanent effects, stop or reduce the medication with your doctor's advice.

Most side effects are 'dose-related'. That is, they may come and go depending on the level of medication you are taking. You may find that a smaller dose relieves the side effect while still helping with the endometriosis.

I'm not very keen on conventional medicine. I've been seeing a homoeopath for years rather than a GP, but my mother insisted on my getting advice for this problem, and it has been diagnosed as endometriosis. The doctor has prescribed danazol, but I'm really not happy and still want to seek homoeopathic advice. Is this wise?

More and more members of the orthodox medical profession are accepting the demonstrable value of many forms of alternative medicine. It doesn't actually matter what anyone else thinks; if it *works* for you, then it must be a wise course to choose. In fact, many practitioners now like to talk in terms of these being 'complementary' rather than 'alternative' therapies. Acupuncture, once considered quackery, has been proved to have value, and is now available on the NHS from many physiotherapists.

So talk to this GP and find out his or her opinion, and follow your own feelings on the matter. Some 300 fully qualified doctors in the UK are also homoeopathic practitioners. As long as your own homoeopath is registered with the Society of Homoeopaths or the British Homoeopathic Association (see the Useful Addresses section of this book) you will be in reliable and ethical hands.

My doctor says that the only way to clear my endometriosis is for me to have a hysterectomy and lose my ovaries. It's not that I want any more children, but I'm terrified of losing my womanhood.

Most women find the idea of a hysterectomy terrifying. We are brought up to see having children as our most important job, and the real proof of our femininity. Once our womb has been taken away, we feel that we will become old, undesirable and useless. Well, that just isn't true. If you need a hysterectomy, the chances are that you will feel healthier, livelier and even sexier, once the operation is over, than you do now.

Most of the problems resulting from hysterectomy are not caused by the operation itself or its after effects, but by our fears and misapprehensions about it. If you go into the operation convinced it will leave you with a pot-belly, grey hair and as much sex appeal as an old sock, then the chances are you won't be in any condition to notice it has done nothing of the sort. And if your partner is so riddled with guilt and unspoken fears that you can't talk about these things, you are both bound to have difficulties. Ask your doctor for more information, and discuss this with him or her and your family. Finally, have a look at the lists at the end of this book for helpful reading on just this subject and for the address of a self-help support group.

I'm in my forties, and our family is complete. My doctor is being very helpful, but I wonder if he is being too cautious. I've tried danazol and found the side effects almost as bad as the problems caused by my endometriosis. I've asked my doctor about having a total hysterectomy, including my ovaries, but he seems to want me to keep on with the more conservative treatments. Should I insist?

Ultimately, your body is your property and your health is your responsibility, but your doctor is behaving correctly in wanting to conserve your ovaries as long as possible. Your own menopause is likely to come in the next five to ten years, and bring with it a resolution of your endometriosis problems. The longer you can keep your ovaries, however, the better protected you will be from the dramatic effects of osteoporosis. This is a condition in which bones lose mass and become brittle in texture due to calcium leaching away. It affects most elderly people to some degree, but is worse in menopausal women since lack of oestrogen encourages the condition.

After the menopause, some 2 to 3 or even 5 per cent of bone mass can be lost each year. So if you have your ovaries removed at forty-five, by the age of fifty-five you may have lost almost a third to a half of your bone mass, which will make you very vulnerable to fractures. So it really is a question of balance and choice. You can minimize the risk of osteoporosis in three ways – by taking Hormone Replacement Therapy (HRT); by taking calcium supplements or increasing the amount of calcium in your diet by consuming more milk, yoghurt and cheese; or by taking regular exercise.

If you stay with the conservative treatments, you may need to live with your endometriosis for another ten years. If not, you gamble on endometriosis not being stimulated by HRT, or on being one of the lucky ones who doesn't react in this way. If you lose this gamble, you will have to choose again whether or not to tolerate the symptoms to benefit from protective effects of the oestrogen in the HRT. Either way, I do recommend that you start on a sensible exercise programme. Whatever you choose, doing vigorous exercise three times a week can only improve your health.

My doctor has booked me a hospital appointment to have an exploratory operation next week. I'm going on holiday in three months' time. Should I buy a one-piece costume to hide the scars, or will I be able to show off in a bikini?

If all you are having is an exploratory, you can confidently get yourself the briefest bikini you can find! You will emerge from the operation with two tiny cuts that may need no more than a couple of stitches or a staple. One of the incisions may well actually be in your navel. Any spectator is going to have to get *awfully* close to see it, and if he's that close, I don't think he will be looking for scars! If there is another incision, it will be lower down, on your tummy. After three months, it will have faded to a faint mark. I don't think that you'll find it attracts notice or looks at all unsightly.

If you are to have more extensive surgery, whether it changes the way you dress on the beach all depends on how much is done to you. You will find that all surgeons are now aware of such concern, and will take pride in leaving you with as neat a scar as possible. Laparotomies, where a slit does have to be made, are usually done below the hair-line, and a brief bikini bottom will easily hide any resulting marks. Even a hysterectomy can be done through such a minimally visible site.

I've had danazol treatment, and reacted dreadfully to it. I've had progestogen, and it didn't work. I've had surgery, and had my womb removed – and the endometriosis came back a few years later! After my experience with danazol, I don't want to try GnRH analogues, so I'm on the combined Pill even though I am forty and it's put my blood pressure up. I just don't seem to be able to find the answer. Any suggestions?

Cultivate a sense of humour – you'll need it! Seriously, endometriosis does seem intractable in some women, and every treatment can give rise to some unpleasant side effect or other. The only option here is to give them a try and settle for the one that gives the largest amount of relief with the smallest amount of discomfort. Then, accept the reality that you are striving for the most bearable, rather than perfection.

You may certainly find that some self-help measures give you much needed support, and I really can highly recommend the benefits of regular exercise in this. You don't have to become an Olympic champion to do yourself some good. Just pick a sport you find fun and that will get you breathing heavily and perspiring – jogging, a keep-fit class, weight-training, swimming, cycling, or even walking – and do it at least three times a week. Once a day is even better, and it really will help with your physical *and* your emotional well-being. Watch your diet, try some of the supplements suggested in Chapter 5, such as Evening Primrose oil, and see how they help you. You may even find that persistence wins in the end!

My mother had a shadow on her lung. It came and went, and puzzled her doctor for years. He freely admits that it was a lucky coincidence that yet another of her 'negative–nothing found' reports from the hospital was on his desk at the same time as a medical magazine with an article on endometriosis. But surely, he should have diagnosed it and sent her to a specialist earlier?

Because endometriosis usually involves tissue normally found in a reproductive organ, and because *most* of the time it affects the same region, your symptoms would normally lead you to seeing either a gynaecologist or an endocrinologist. A gynaecologist is a specialist in diseases of the female reproductive system, and an endocrinologist is expert in hormones and hormone-producing glands. The average ears, nose and throat, chest, or skin specialist may not know enough about endometriosis (or not remember what he or she was taught in medical school) to connect the symptoms that led to your being sent to him or her to this rather obscure variation of the disease. Researchers are now suggesting that endometriosis should not be thought of as a purely gynaecological condition, but as a systemic one. That is, a disease that can affect the body as a whole, rather than being located and confined to one area or one organ.

I've been told I have endometriosis and that I should take drugs to get rid of it. The only thing that really worries me is that if these drugs will kill all traces of endometriosis in my body, won't they also get rid of the lining of my womb? How will I be able to get pregnant afterwards?

Medical therapy, whether it is danazol, a GnRH analogue, oestrogen/progestogen or progestogen-only, works against endometriosis but leaves the lining of your womb still functional. The reason for this is that ectopic, or 'outside the womb', endometriotic tissue does not behave in *exactly* the same way as entopic, or inside the womb, endometrial tissue.

When you take such treatments, the tissue inside the womb *will* atrophy or waste away at the same time as endometriotic tissue elsewhere. But the ectopic tissue also regresses and is absorbed. That is, its roots die out as well, leaving no remains from which to start growing again. It is usually found that if endometriosis returns in a woman who has successfully completed a course of treatment, it does not strike in the same area again, but attacks new sites. However, the actual lining of the womb itself, the endometrium, still has its base, and once a treatment is stopped it will go back to growing again as normal.

I would like to get pregnant as soon as possible, but at the moment my doctor is treating me for endometriosis. Should I wait until this treatment is over before trying for a baby? If so, how soon can I then try?

It all depends on the treatment. Some treatments will positively stop your getting pregnant. If you are on combined oestrogen and progestogen therapy or on progestogen therapy, it is highly unlikely that you will conceive. The usual advice we give is for women to wait some months after coming off this type of treatment before they try for a pregnancy. This is *not* because the pills will leave a residue in the body that could be passed to and harm the baby. In fact, the substances in the pills pass out of the body quite quickly, and this is why a woman can fall pregnant *immediately* after she comes off the Pill.

The reason for the suggested delay is that your body can still take a few weeks or months to get its own hormonal rhythm back, and it is common to miss a period, or even two, after the immediate withdrawal bleed that follows once you have taken your last Pill. If you try for a baby at once, *this* missed period may be mistaken for the first missed period of a pregnancy, and you then may be weeks or even months out when trying to calculate the exact age of a developing foetus. This may not seem to matter, but it is sometimes hard to calculate this age by examination or any other means. If your doctors then think you have come to term, and induce what they think is a two-week late baby, when it is in fact only thirty-eight or even thirty-six weeks, you and your baby could be in trouble.

If you are on danazol, it is vital that you don't get pregnant, since if your baby is female, the medication could make her have some masculine characteristics. Danazol in itself should stop any possibility of a pregnancy, but there are rare reports of this happening, and so you should use barrier contraception as well during your period of treatment. Again, the effects of this therapy pass fairly quickly, but waiting a month or so would be helpful. Basically, the best advice is to *tell* your doctor you want to become pregnant, *ask* for his or her advice and then follow it.

I'm twenty-six, and have just been diagnosed as having mild endometriosis. What should I do? Does this mean I will never be able to have children?

Not necessarily. Endometriosis and infertility seem to have an association, but they don't always go hand in hand. Your best course would be to make sure your endometriosis is treated, even though it is mild. No one should ever *assume* they are going to have children – children are far too difficult and responsible a task to just take on without proper consideration. So you should have a long think about whether you really want a child, and *why*, before going any further. If yours is a genuine, mature and deeply felt decision, then you may have to start considering it seriously soon.

It certainly appears that endometriosis sufferers are most successful in their attempts to get pregnant in the first year after treatment, and get steadily less so from two years after treatment.

So, all things being equal, you might want to spend the next six months or so on treatment, and then concentrate on trying for a baby. If after a year of trying (and remember, it can take even a normally fertile couple this long to succeed) there is still no pregnancy, you still have ample time to seek specialist infertility advice and treatment. Tell the doctors who are treating you for your endometriosis that pregnancy *is* on your mind, and discuss it further with them.

I am receiving treatment for endometriosis, and most of the symptoms that made life so unpleasant are getting better. One of my worries, of course, is that after four years of trying, we have still not had a baby. If once I finish the treatment all is well, can I then expect to get pregnant?

The experience of many endometriosis sufferers *is* that successful treatment of other symptoms can lead to pregnancy as well. However, it should be noted that research on endometriosis does not give a clear-cut picture. This is why it is suggested that infertility might cause endometriosis, rather than the other way round. It could even be that both the infertility and the endometriosis are caused by a third factor. Depending on the nature of your case, you may need to tackle the root cause of infertility or the third factor, as well as deal with the endometriosis, before being sure that a pregnancy is possible. Talk to your doctor about this. It may be necessary for you to be seen by the appropriate specialist, with infertility specifically in mind, as well as being seen for your endometriosis.

I finished my treatment for endometriosis six months ago, and I'm delighted to say I'm now pregnant. However, I'm worried in case my endometriosis puts me at a higher risk of having a miscarriage.

Several reports have suggested that women with endometriosis suffer an increased number of miscarriages. These studies also seem to show that the rate falls after treatment. However, a more recent and more scientific study questioned these findings. The thinking now is that although, theoretically, infertility can be caused in women with endometriosis by a reaction between her body and an embryo that results in spontaneous abortion, as yet we have no conclusive proof that these abortions happen more in endometriosis patients than with anyone else.

We do know that high stress can increase your risk of spontaneous abortion, so the best advice is not to worry. This is a bit like telling you that you will inherit a fortune as long as you walk past the next cat you see without thinking of its tail (try it!). Try taking up yoga, do keep-fit, demand hourly massages from your mate, think beautiful thoughts, stroke a cat – anything that will bring your stress levels down. And stop worrying.

I was diagnosed as having endometriosis three years ago, and I've had treatment off and on ever since. We've been trying for a baby for just over a year now. A friend has suggested that, since other treatments haven't worked, we should try for a test-tube baby. Would this be possible?

You could certainly try. Women whose infertility is associated with endometriosis are now being accepted on to IVF, or *in-vitro* (literally, 'in glass') fertilization, programmes. However, it does seem that women with endometriosis have a lesser chance of success in giving birth this way than women who are infertile for other reasons.

In *in-vitro* fertilization, women are given treatment – usually clomiphene citrate (trade name Clomid) – to stimulate the ovaries into producing several mature eggs at the same time. The woman is monitored by ultrasound to pinpoint when the follicles will burst open. As the time approaches, a fine needle is passed through the abdominal wall and the ripe eggs are aspirated or sucked out. They are then mixed in a dish – the 'glass' – with sperm. When fertilization has taken place, several routes may then be taken.

The developing bundle of cells can be put back directly into the womb, having been kept in the laboratory for several days to simulate the time it would otherwise have taken to travel down the Fallopian tube. If this was not done, it would be in the womb at too early a stage in its development to be able to implant properly. Experience has shown that if only one embryo is placed in the womb, its chances of survival are far lower than if several are put in at the same time. The optimum number to insert is now agreed to be four, and in most cases where the procedure succeeds, one or two will go on to develop fully. In some cases, three or four will do so, which is why 'test tube' treatment does carry the risk of causing multiple births.

More recently, it has been found that putting the fertilized egg back into the body at an earlier stage at the entrance to the Fallopian tubes and allowing it to be wafted into the tubes and carried down increases the chances of success. The embryo seems to respond better to this more 'natural' approach, and only one embryo is needed. This procedure is known as GIFT or gamete intrafallopian transfer.

The problems associated with endometriosis are varied. It seems that women with the condition have more difficulty in producing eggs, even under the stimulation of Clomid, especially if they have severe endometriosis. Furthermore, if their pelvis has adhesions or their abdomen has operation scars, the ultrasound operator may have difficulties telling if and when the ovaries are producing ripe follicles. Adhesions on or around the Fallopian tubes may obviously put a barrier in the way of an embryo, or the cilia inside the tubes may have a limited ability to wave the embryo on its way.

It has also been noticed that even when eggs *are* collected from endometriosis sufferers, they seem to become fertilized less often than those from women with other causes of infertility. However, when the eggs of a woman with endometriosis are successfully fertilized, they continue on to the next stage of development normally *in vitro*. When GIFT is used with endometriosis patients, the embryo may not develop any further. Some factor in the fluid found in the pelvic cavity and the Fallopian tubes is likely to be to blame. Once the embryo has implanted in the womb, endometriosis patients are still at risk, since spontaneous abortion rates seem to be higher than among other women.

Is it therefore worthwhile? IVF and GIFT are expensive procedures in terms of money, time and emotion. They are available in some places, and to some patients, on the National Health Service, but the heavy commitment of people and resources means that availability *is* limited. Going private is an option. However, one cycle of treatment (that is, treatment leading up to one attempt at implanting an embryo) could cost up to several thousand pounds, and success rates are often counted in terms of 5 to 10 per cent a cycle.

One thing does seem to emerge. Success at achieving a pregnancy in women with endometriosis is most likely in the first year of receiving conventional treatment, and very low after two years. After three years, if you haven't yet become pregnant, your best chances are likely to be with IVF or GIFT, but even these chances *are* low. It may be a good idea for you and your husband to start considering how you would cope with a life without your own children. There *are* other options, however bleak or unlikely they can seem at the moment.

I can't believe our luck, but I've fallen pregnant on only my first IVF treatment – I understand that's unusually good going. However, I seem to remember someone saying that endometriosis patients have a greater risk of having a miscarriage after IVF. Is this true?

What some researchers have said is that eggs collected from endometriosis patients have less than half the chance of fertilizing *in vitro* than those collected from other infertile women. In fact, they put your chances of achieving fertilization at one in three. A few studies have also come up with higher than normal rates of spontaneous abortion in women with advanced endometriosis.

If your endometriosis *was* severe, you may well have to be

prepared for disappointment. The evidence seems to point to spontaneous abortions happening quite early on in pregnancy if they are going to happen at all. So, once you are safely into your second trimester, you should be able to relax.

CHAPTER EIGHT

What Can You Do?

Having read – or glanced through – this book, what are your options now? You might be in one of three situations at the moment:

1. You *don't* have endometriosis, but wonder whether you may be at risk of developing it in the future. Is there anything you can do to minimize your chances?
2. You have some, or many, of the symptoms described in Chapter 3. How can you find out if endometriosis *is* your problem, and what can you do then?
3. You have been diagnosed, and are somewhere along the treatment route. What now?

What can *you* do at each stage to make life better for yourself?

As a woman who does not have endometriosis, you can:

THINK SAFE SEX

If, as some evidence suggests, endometriosis can be encouraged by a case of PID, you can make absolutely sure that you do not catch a sexually transmitted disease or allow one to develop past its early stages. Since some conditions, notably gonorrhoea, can be symptomless in many cases, the best form of attack is a good defence. Until you are totally sure that your sexual partner is *not* infected and is not having another relationship (and has not had one for some time), use a condom and spermicide. Most spermicides that are now available contain an ingredient called nonoxynol-9 which not only kills sperm to protect you from a pregnancy, but also destroys many of the elements that could give you an STD.

Be choosey about your relationships, but remember that like any other illness, STDs can be caught and passed on by the squeaky-clean boy or girl next door just as easily as by the unsavoury and the promiscuous. Outward charm and appearance are no guide to whether or not your lover is going to put you at risk! And if you do feel you might have been at risk, go along to a Sexually Transmitted Disease Clinic *at once* for a check up.

THINK HORMONES

Consider carefully whether you are going to have children at all and, if so, at what time in your life. In many cases, late childbearing is the best *social* option (that is, a child born by choice to parents who have a proven strong relationship and a good financial base). It is far from easy to build up your marriage, your home and your job or career *and* make the enormous adjustments needed to welcome a baby, all at the same time. Couples who have a child in their mid or late twenties, or in their thirties, are more likely to find their greater maturity and confidence a distinct asset.

Physically, statistics suggest that the optimum time for childbirth is likely to be the mid to late twenties. Most illnesses, or death in both babies and mothers occur less often at this time than in a teenage or much later pregnancy. However, leaving it to your late twenties can increase your risk of endometriosis either developing or worsening. You may need to weigh up a whole parcel of ethical, practical, emotional and financial considerations before arriving at a decision that suits you.

If you are going to delay childbearing until fairly late in life, consider using artificial hormones to substitute for the protective effects of pregnancy and lactation. We often deride the Pill on the grounds that it isn't 'natural' to put all those artificial chemicals into our bodies. The problem is that having a gap of ten to twenty years between starting periods and having a first baby is far from 'natural' either.

Animals and humans have evolved ensuring the continuation of the species by reproducing regularly. To make up for all those members of the tribe lost to starvation, disease and sabre-toothed tigers, early woman was *meant* to get pregnant and to have new babies every year or so until her natural death at the age of about thirty. We, of course, don't live in this 'natural' state any more. Few Western women die of starvation, most disease is under control and the sabre-toothed tiger has suffered the fate of most things that got in the way of our species. Better nutrition and a lower pregnancy rate has doubled our life expectancy, which means that if we want to preserve that life in all its unnatural glory, it is not logical to draw a line and say, 'I'll accept the help of technology up to *this* point, but no further.'

Using hormones to mimic a pregnant state is hardly 'putting something foreign into your body'. What it does is mimic the *natural* state you might otherwise be in if you lived in the primitive society your body is designed to inhabit. So, consider using an oral contraceptive, not just to stop ovulation and prevent pregnancy, but also to limit the number of times your endometrium builds and sheds in the space of a year. Evidence suggests that it is healthier – and, dare I say it, more natural – to use the Pill continuously and have only four or two periods each year. To achieve this take four or nine packets consecutively before having a week off to allow a period. You can then resume for a further four or nine packets. This can be done with any of the combined oral contraceptive Pills, except the bi- or tri-phasic Pills.

These include two or three different strengths of Pill through the three-week course. You can recognize them by the fact that the pills will be in two or three different colours in each packet, rather than the single colour of the ordinary combined Pill. Since the pills at the end and the beginning of each pack are of very different strengths, going straight from one packet to another will cause a sudden drop in hormone levels, and may well trigger ovulation, ruining the whole point of the exercise. So, if you do want to try this idea, you need to ask your doctor to prescribe another type of Pill to use as a 'sandwich', and then take this for a week in between each packet of bi- or tri-phasic Pills. Needless to say, if you do want to use your Pill in this way, you must discuss it with your doctor. Quite apart from the fact that he or she should be aware of what you are doing and why, you will need to have extra packets of Pills. If you leave the usual seven-day break in between each packet, you only use thirteen in a year – one every four weeks. If you take them without a break you will need sixteen to eighteen packets a year. If you are one of the women for whom the combined Pill may represent health risks, consider the progestogen-only, or 'mini', Pill. This, too, is likely to protect you from endometriosis.

As a woman who has some of the symptoms of endometriosis you can:

THINK SELF-CONFIDENCE

Your first port of call will be your own doctor. You may have a doctor you trust and with whom you get on. On the other hand, you may be unlucky enough to have a distant or prickly relationship, especially if your symptoms have led to a series of unsatisfactory encounters with the medical profession – and your own doctor in particular – in the past. Whatever, go to *this* consultation with a fresh point of view. Trust yourself for having a good reason for making this visit, and don't allow yourself to sabotage the proceedings by being apologetic or vague. *Write down* the symptoms that have prompted your being there, and the worries and questions you have about your problems. If your doctor does not mention endometriosis, ask about it yourself. If your doctor does not suggest seeing a specialist, do so yourself. Be polite, but firm. You *know* something is wrong, and you would like your doctor's professional help to do something about it. In the unhappy, and thankfully uncommon, situation where a doctor is unable to give you a satisfactory explanation for your difficulties and to offer proper help, and is unwilling to send you for further examination and treatment, take your custom elsewhere.

As a woman who has endometriosis, you can:

THINK HEALTH

As has been already discussed, we are just beginning to understand the power of mind over body. Mental attitudes can affect the production of chemical substances in our brains and bodies. These, in turn, can push us towards ill heath or well-being. Those dealing with cancer sufferers and men and women who have contracted HIV – the virus that can lead to AIDS – appear to have produced extraordinary results with therapy that involves thinking oneself into a state of well-being. Sufferers are encouraged to use 'imaging', a process in which they picture their own immune system fighting back against disease, and to use willpower to make their body win against 'invaders', or the tissue that has betrayed and turned against them. By raising our self-confidence and self-esteem and by telling ourselves we *will* be healthy and we *will* be well, many of us can achieve exactly what we desire. Self-help groups of people in the same situation can be enormously helpful, as they provide encouragement and mutual support in low moments.

THINK FLEXIBLE

Since endometriosis is such a mysterious disease and we know so little about its development and cure, it makes sense to consider every remedy we can lay our hands on. If you trust orthodox medicine, that is no reason to dismiss the possible benefits of Evening Primrose oil, selenium or acupuncture. All have been found to increase the action of other conventional therapies when taken in conjunction with them. Obviously, keep your doctor informed, and also keep within the guidelines given for any of the alternative therapies. Overdosing on selenium or vitamin B6 *is* as unwise and dangerous as overdosing on any prescribed medicine would be.

Listen to what other endometriosis sufferers have tried. If it has worked for them, however strange and unconventional it might seem, see if it will work for you. Keep an open mind to every idea but one – that endometriosis is incurable and you may as well lie down and let it defeat you. That is *not* an option!

THINK INFORMATION

Keep yourself informed. Joining a self-help group and making friends with your doctor are good ways of doing this. Until you find a solution, keep badgering your medical advisers as to whether anything new is available that you could try. If you keep on top of the subject, you know that you are in control of your endometriosis, rather than letting your endometriosis take control of you and your life.

DON'T JUST THINK HEALTH, DO IT!

Above all, and whatever stage you are at, seize life with both hands and make yours a vigorous and joyful lifestyle. Look at the food you eat and make it as delicious *and* as healthy a diet as possible. Give your body the best building blocks to make you bouncy and glowing – fresh fruit; fresh vegetables; fish and chicken; lean meat; low-fat milk, cheese, yoghurts and spreads; wholewheat cereals, breads and pasta. And remember that cakes, biscuits, cream, sweets and jams are for deserved treats, not for every meal. There is nothing boring, difficult or even exhausting about producing meals that taste and look good, and *do* you good. It just means breaking some old bad habits and taking up good new ones.

Another bad habit to break is the no-exercise one. You do not have to starve yourself to achieve a good figure. All you have to do is to take vigorous exercise three times a week, and the difference can be amazing. The big surprise about exercise is that it is far more fun and far less tiring than sitting slumped doing nothing. Getting yourself hot and sweaty actually perks up the system and you feel livelier and *more* invigorated after a session than when you began. And it is hardly unfeminine or degrading to get into that sort of state when some of the world's most influential and beautiful women do it regularly. Doing keep-fit, jogging, badminton or squash, or even walking can help strengthen your bones, melt away fat, and kill pain – useful, whether you are an endometriosis sufferer or not.

A final word

There is life both with and after endometriosis. It may be true that one in every two sufferers who receive treatment goes on to have a recurrence. But look at that another way: half of the women who seek help *do* emerge free of the disease. Your worst enemy is not the disease and not the medical profession, even if they have let you down so far. Your worst enemy is passivity. Passivity allows you to give in to pressure and not pursue a diagnosis or treatment. Passivity allows you to sit back and let *them* try to cure you, with no input from yourself. Passivity allows intractable endometriosis to become the ruling factor of our lives.

Endometriosis will be beaten on a large scale when doctors understand it and find out how to deal with it. The more patients they have battering down their doors and demanding a solution, the more incentive there will be to research this condition. And endometriosis will be beaten on an individual scale when *we*, the endo sufferers, seize the disease by the scruff of the neck and refuse to let it take control over how we feel, how we love and how we act.

Further Reading

Understanding endometriosis

Coping with Endometriosis, Dr Lyle Breitkopf and Marion Gordon Bakoulis, Grapevine, 1988.
> Helpful information and advice by two American authors.

Endometriosis: Contemporary Concepts in Clinical Management, ed. Robert S. Schenken, Lippincott, 1989.
> A detailed and comprehensive review of the clinical aspects of endometriosis. Written for doctors and very technical, but worth struggling through.

Functional Disorders of the Menstrual Cycle, M. G. Bush and E. M. Goudsmit, Wiley, 1988.
> As above, another medical text covering many disorders of the menstrual cycle. Includes two very useful chapters on endometriosis. Again, written for doctors but worth struggling through.

Overcoming Endometriosis, Mary Lou Ballweg and Susan Deutsch, Arlington Books, 1987.
> Written by the American Endometriosis Association, with a foreword by the British Endometriosis Association. A detailed volume that lists many research papers.

Understanding Endometriosis, Caroline Hawkridge, Optima, 1989.
> Published in conjunction with the National Endometriosis Society, it gives a straightforward account of diagnosis and the varying attitudes of the medical profession. It discusses the physical and psychological effects of endometriosis, and what treatments are available.

Research and medical papers

There are literally hundreds of research papers, going back to von Rokitansky in 1860 and up to the most recent. Probably all those published before 1989 are listed in *Endometriosis: Contemporary Concepts in Clinical Management*. Medical journals such as the *British Medical Journal*, the *Lancet*, the *British Journal of Obstetrics and Gynaecology*, the *Journal of the American Medical Association*, and many others will have published more since then. The British Library will have them on file, and you can obtain any you need through inter-library loans via your own local library.

More about your body and some specific problems

The Amarant Book of HRT, Teresa Gorman and Dr Malcolm Whitehead, Pan Books, 1989.
> Explains how HRT can reduce symptoms of the menopause and protect against osteoporosis.

Avoiding Osteoporosis, Dr Allan Dixon and Dr Anthony Woolf, Optima, 1987.
> Explains the different treatments available, including HRT.

Brittle Bones and the Calcium Crisis, Kathleen Mayes, Thorsons, 1987.
> Information on osteoporosis and how to fight it.

Candida Albicans – Can Yeast be Your Problem?, Leon Chaitow, Thorsons, 1985.
> All about candida, and the wide variety of problems it can cause – depression, diarrhoea and menstrual difficulties – as well as thrush.

Coping with Periods, Dr Diana Sanders, Chambers, 1985.
> Practical help and advice on periods and their problems and how to deal with them.

Coping with Thrush, Caroline Clayton, Sheldon Press, 1984.
> Sensitive and practical explanations and advice on controlling the
> infection both with medical and self-help remedies. Useful
> checklist of dos and don'ts.

Cystitis, Dr Kathryn Schrotenboer and Sue Berkman, Optima,
1987.
> A comprehensive approach to cystitis and its treatments.

Hysterectomy: What it is and How to Cope with it Successfully,
Suzie Hayman, Sheldon Press, 1986.
> A detailed guide which explains why an operation may be needed,
> and what to expect from your doctors and in hospital. It also
> discusses your emotional and physical state before and after the
> operation.

Menopause, Raewyn Mackenzie, Thorsons, 1984.
> An honest self-help book with a positive approach.

Menopause: A Guide for Women of All Ages, Jill Rakusen, National
Extension College, 1989.
> An unbiased discussion of all aspects of the menopause and how
> to prevent osteoporosis.

Menopause: The Natural Way, Dr Sadja Greenwood, Optima, 1987.
> A positive approach to the middle years. Covers HRT, health care
> and post-menopausal sexuality.

Understanding Cystitis, Angela Kilmartin, Century Arrow, 1985.
> Two books by the 'guru' of cystitis, brought together in a new
> volume and offering sound and proven help to cystitis sufferers.

Understanding Premenstrual Tension, Dr Michael Bush, Pan,
Books, 1984.
> Approachable, sympathetic, understandable and practical advice
> from one of the leading experts in this field.

The Well Woman Handbook: A Guide to Women throughout their Lives, Suzie Hayman, Penguin Books, 1989.

> A comprehensive guide to the female reproductive system and what can go wrong; self-examination techniques and contraception.

Alternative – or Complementary – Medicine

Alternative Health Care for Women, Patsy Westcott, Thorsons, 1987.

> Discusses common health problems as well as fertility and reproduction. Focuses on preventive health care and has informative sections on different therapies.

Alternative Medicine, Dr Anthony Stanway, Penguin Books, 1986.

> A detailed guide to natural therapies, listing thirty-two different disciplines from acupuncture to yoga, via aromatherapy, naturopathy, psionic healing and rolfing.

Aromatherapy for Everyone, Robert Tisserand, Penguin Books, 1988.

> Explains what aromatherapy is, how it developed and how it can help you.

Curing PMT the Drug-Free Way, Moira Carpenter, Century, 1985.

> A self-help guide to understanding PMT and its relief through diet, homoeopathy, herbal remedies and relaxation techniques.

Herbal Medicine for Everyone, Michael McIntyre, Penguin Books, 1988.

> How the modern herbalist works, and what treatment can be offered to you by a qualified herbal doctor.

Homoeopathic Medicine at Home, Maesimund B. Panos and Jane Heimlich, Corgi, 1980.

> A comprehensive and practical guide to the theory and use of homoeopathic remedies.

Coping with Stress and Depression

Anxiety and Depression – a Practical Guide to Recovery, Prof. Robert Priest, Optima, 1983.

An explanation of the causes of depression and anxiety, and a practical guide to self-help and getting professional assistance.

Coming Off Tranquillizers, Shirley Trickett, Thorsons, 1986.
Step by step guide to coming off tranquillizers, with an honest explanation of what may happen and how to cope.

Coping with Stress, Dr G. Wilkinson, BMA (Family Doctor), 1987.
Explains what stress is and the problems it creates. Advice on self-help and sources of further assistance.

Depression and its Treatment, John Hinton, BMA (Family Doctor), 1986.
Explains what depression is, common causes, where to seek help and the varieties of treatment.

The Magic of Massage, Ouida West, Century, 1983.
A comprehensive guide to the many techniques of massage – from how to do a quick self-massage to giving the complete sixty-minute body massage. Information also on acupuncture, shiatsu, herbs and meditation.

Massage and Loving, Anne Hooper, Unwin Hyman, 1988.
Shows how simple massage can relieve tension for family and friends, or how erotic massage can be shared with lovers.

Stresswise, Dr Terry Looker and Dr Olga Gregson, Hodder and Stoughton, 1989.
A practical guide to understanding and dealing with stress.

Super Massage, Gordon Inkeles, Piatkus Books, 1989.
Step by step instructions to massage techniques that can turn pain into pleasure and reduce stress.

Women and Depression, Deidre Sanders, Sheldon Press, 1984.
Positive guide to what triggers depression and what you can do about it.

Women and Tranquillizers, Celia Haddon, Sheldon Press, 1984.
> Describes the different types of tranquillizers and explains why you might have been given them, what they do, their possible side effects and how to come off using them.

Building self-esteem and tackling sexual problems.

I'm OK, you're OK, Thomas A. Harris, Pan Books, 1973.
> Aims to get you in control of yourself, your relationships and your future – no matter what has happened in your past.

Making the Most of Loving, Gill Cox and Sheila Dainow, Sheldon Press, 1988.
> An understanding guide to all aspects of love and sex – how your body works, how to be a good lover and what to do if things go wrong.

Making the Most of Yourself, Gill Cox and Sheila Dainow, Sheldon Press, 1985.
> A straightforward guide to self-improvement and problem-solving. Aims to increase your confidence, self-awareness and control.

Sex Problems, Martin Cole and Wendy Dryden, Optima, 1989.
> The facts about sex, sex problems and sex therapy. Written in an easily readable style by two experienced therapists.

Treat Yourself to Sex, Paul Brown and Carolyn Faulder, Penguin Books, 1988.
> A readable and sympathetic handbook that deals with a range of common sexual problems.

A Woman in Your Own Right, Anne Dickson, Quartet, 1985.
> The classic book on the method of assertiveness training to help women learn to handle personal, social, sexual and professional situations.

Women and Sex, Anne Hooper, Sheldon Press, 1986.
> Clear, objective and understanding guide to common sexual problems and what to do about them. Includes a comprehensive list of helping agencies.

Pursuing a healthy lifestyle.

Safer Sex: A New Look at Sexual Pleasure, Peter Gordon and Louise Mitchell, Faber & Faber, 1988.
>As well as being a guide to safe sex, this book also examines our attitudes to sex and sexuality.

Sunday Times ABC Diet and Bodyplan, Oliver Gillie and Susana Raby, Hutchinson, 1984.
>For the overweight, overstressed and out of condition, a comprehensive gimmick-free eight-week programme for getting fit, losing weight and building a healthy lifestyle.

Infertility and its treatments

Adoption and Fostering: A Practical Guide, Alison King, Crowood Press, 1989.
>Considers the emotional, financial, legal and practical implications of taking on someone else's child.

Coping with Childlessness, Diane and Peter Houghton, Unwin Hyman, 1987.
>Informative book based on the authors' own experiences, with emphasis on the emotional needs of the childless.

The Gift of a Child, Robert and Elizabeth Snowdon, Unwin Hyman, 1984.
>Explains the male reproductive system, infertility and its treatments, and insemination by donor (AID). Also examines the need for a change in social attitudes, improved facilities and more research.

Hidden Loss: Miscarriage and Ectopic Pregnancy, Valerie Hey, The Women's Press, 1989.
>Information about the known causes of pre-birth loss. Discusses bereavement and mourning and self-help techniques to aid the healing process.

Infertility and In Vitro Fertilization, Dr Leila Hanna and Dr Elliot Philipp, BMA (Family Doctor), 1987.
> Outlines the various causes of infertility and the treatments available, particularly IVF.

Infertility: A Sympathetic Approach, Dr Robert Winston, Optima, 1986.
> Discusses the emotional and ethical issues and tells childless couples how to ensure they receive all the relevant tests.

The Infertility Handbook, Sarah J. Biggs, Fertility Services Management, 1989.
> A privately published handbook by a health professional who is herself on an IVF programme. As well as covering all the facts about infertility and its diagnosis and treatments, it lists NHS and private clinics offering treatment. The book is only available by direct order from Fertility Services Management, The New House, Far End, Sheepscombe, Stroud GL6 7RL (£3.60 inc. p. & p.).

In Search of Parenthood: Coping with Infertility and High-Tech Conception, Judith N. Lasker and Susan Borg, Pandora Press, 1989.
> Discussion of AID, IVF, surrogate motherhood, ovum transfer and donors.

Miscarriage, Margaret Leroy, Optima, 1988.
> What happens when you miscarry, what the causes are, and how you and your partner may feel. How to give your next pregnancy every chance of success.

Why Children?, eds. Stephanie Dowrick and Sibyl Grundberg, The Women's Press, 1980.
> Eighteen women talk honestly and fully about why they chose to have their own children, to adopt children, or not to have children at all. Explores the pleasures and pains of all these options and helps the readers' efforts to understand and make such choices for themselves.

Most of the books listed above would be available from The Family Planning Association Bookshop and through their Mail Order Service 'Healthwise', 27–35 Mortimer Street, London WIN 7RJ, or from Relate, Herbert Gray College, Little Church Street, Rugby, CV21 3AP.

Useful Addresses

There are lots of groups and organizations ready to help you with *any* problem. Some will have a local office near you, and you can use your own telephone phone book to look them up:

COMMUNITY HEALTH COUNCIL
If you have any complaint about the medical profession or need advice about your health.

FAMILY PRACTITIONER COMMITTEE
If you want to change your doctor or are having trouble doing so, or if you have a serious complaint against your GP.

SEXUALLY TRANSMITTED DISEASE, OR 'SPECIAL', CLINIC
Most hospitals have one. They will see you without a referral letter from your own doctor, and will keep your visit private if you insist. Often listed in telephone books under 'VD'.

SAMARITANS
If you really feel down and have no one else to talk to. Look them up in your phone book, or just ask the operator to put you through.

The groups and organizations listed on the following pages often have London addresses. If you live elsewhere, this *doesn't* mean there is no help in your area. Contact the main address and they will be able to put you in touch with your nearest help.

More information on endometriosis

Endometriosis Society
65 Holmdene Avenue
London SE24 6LD
Tel: 071-737 4764 (evenings)

>*Support and self-help for endometriosis sufferers.*
>*Newsletter.*

Women's health and specific problems

Family Planning Association
27–35 Mortimer Street
London WIN 7RJ
Tel: 071-636 7866

>*Free information and leaflets on many aspects of family*
>*planning and reproductive health.*

Health Education Authority
Hamilton House
Mabledon Place
London WC1H 9TX
Tel: 071-631 0930

>*Free information and leaflets on a wide range of health*
>*topics. 'Guide to healthy eating' and 'Exercise, why bother?'*
>*are particularly good.*

Health Promotion Authority for Wales
8th Floor
Brunel House
Fitzallen Place
Cardiff CF2 1EB
Tel: 022-472472

>*Provides the same help as HEA, for Wales.*

Hysterectomy Support Group
c/o WHRRIC
52–4 Featherstone Street
London ECIY 8RT

> *Self-help groups for women having, or who have had,
> hysterectomies.*

Marie Stopes House
The Well Woman Centre
108 Whitfield Street
London WIP 6BE
Tel: 071-388 0662

> *Advice and practical help on all aspects of women's health.
> Well Woman care. Fees charged.*

Menopause Collective
c/o WHRRIC
52–4 Featherstone Street
London ECIY 8RT

> *Information and workshops on the menopause and women's
> self-image.*

**National Association for
Premenstrual Syndrome**
PO Box 72
Sevenoaks TNI3 3PS
Tel: 0732-459378

> *Free information on PMS.*

National Osteoporosis Society
Barton Meade House
PO Box 10
Radstock
Bath BA3 3YB
Tel: 0761-32472

> *Leaflets and newsletter.*

Northern Ireland Health Promotion Unit
23 Hampton Place
Belfast BT7 3JN
Tel: 0232-644811

> *Provides the same help as HEA, for Northern Ireland.*

Pelvic Inflammatory Disease Group
61 Jenner Road
London N16 7RB

> *Support group for women suffering from PID.*

Prem Soc
PO Box 102
London SE1 7ES

> *Can put you in touch with help for PMS in your area.*

Scottish Health Education Group
Health Education Centre
Canaan Lane
Edinburgh EH10 4SG
Tel: 031-447 8044

> *Provides the same help as the HEA, for Scotland.*

TRANX
25a Masons Avenue
Wealdstone
Harrow HA3 5AH
Tel: 081-427 2065/2827

> *Advice and support for tranquillizer users. Leaflets.*

Women's Health and Reproductive Rights Information Centre
52-4 Featherstone Street
London EC1Y 8RT
Tel: 071-251 6580 (11am–5pm Mon. to Fri. except Thurs.)

> *National information and support centre on women's health issues. Contact with self-help groups and publications.*

The Women's Nutritional Advisory Service
PO Box 268
Brighton BN3 1RW
Tel: 0273-771366

> *Advice and information on diet and nutrition for general
> health problems, including PMS. Fees charged.*

Alternative medicine

British Acupuncture Association and Register
34 Alderney Street
London SW1V 4EU
Tel: 071-834 1012

> *Can put you in touch with a registered practitioner.*

British Herbal Medicine Association
The Old Coach House
Southborough Road
Surbiton
Surrey

> *Information and advice on herbal medicine.*

British Holistic Medical Association
179 Gloucester Place
London NW1 6DX
Tel: 071-262 5299

> *Information for doctors and general public on holistic
> medicine. Reading lists and addresses and leaflets.*

British Homoeopathic Association
27a Devonshire Street
London W1N 1RJ

> *Information on homoeopathy, including how to find an
> NHS practitioner.*

British Naturopathic and Osteopathic College and Clinic
6 Netherhall Gardens
London NW3 5RR

> *Information on therapies and clinics.*

Institute for Complementary Medicine
21 Portland Place
London WIN 3AF

> *Information on a wide range of alternative therapies.*

National Institute of Medical Herbalists
41 Hatherley Road
Winchester SO22 6RR

> *Can put you in touch with a herbalist.*

Society of Homoeopaths
2 Artizan Road
Northampton NNI 4HU
Tel: 0604-21400

> *Can put you in touch with a private homoeopathic practitioner.*

General advice and support

Association of Community Health Councils
30 Drayton Park
London N5 IPB
Tel: 071-609 8405

> *Can put you in touch with your nearest CHC.*

British Association for Counselling
37a Sheep Street
Rugby CV21 3BX
Tel: 0788-78328

> *Information on counselling services.*

Citizens Advice Bureau (CAB)
Myddelton House
115–23 Pentonville Road
London NI 9LS
Tel: 071-833 2181

> *Free advice on any subject.*

Institute of Psychosexual Medicine
11 Chandos Street
London WIM OEB
Tel: 071-580 1043

> *Trains therapists and can put you in touch with a local practitioner.*

Patients Association
Room 33
18 Charing Cross Road
London WC2H OHR
Tel: 071-240 0671

> *Help and advice on any question relating to patient care.*

Relate (National Marriage Guidance)
Herbert Gray College
Little Church Street
Rugby CV21 3AP
Tel: 0788-73241

> *Counselling for problems in relationships.*

Women's Therapy Centre
6 Manor Gardens
London N7 6LA
Tel: 071-263 6200

> *Trains therapists and runs courses and workshops for women on a wide range of women's problems. Fees charged.*

Infertility

British Agencies for Adoption and Fostering
11 Southwark Street
London SE1 1RQ
Tel: 071-407 8800

> *Information and support on any aspect of adoption or fostering. Helpful leaflets and booklets.*

Miscarriage Association
PO Box 24
Ossett WF5 9XG
Tel: 0924-830515

> *Information and support.*

National Association for the Childless
318 Summer Lane
Birmingham B19 3RL
Tel: 021-359 4887

> *Self-help organization for people with fertility problems. Advice, counselling and regional contacts.*

Parent to Parent Information on Adoption Services
Lower Boddington
Daventry NN11 6YB
Tel: 0327-60295

> *Self-help support and information service for adoptive and prospective adoptive families.*

Pregnancy Advisory Service
13 Charlotte Street
London WIP 1HD
Tel: 071-637 8962

> *Information, counselling and practical assistance with infertility and psychosexual problems. Fees charged.*

Stillbirth and Neo-natal Death Society
28 Falkland Place
London wim 4de
Tel: 071-436 5881

> *Information and support.*

Getting healthy, staying healthy

Action on Smoking and Health (ASH)
5–11 Mortimer Street
London win 7rh
Tel: 071-637 9843

> *Information service and pressure group offering free
> literature on smoking and health.*

BPAS (British Pregnancy Advisory Service)
Austy Manor
Wootton Wawen
Solihull b95 6da
Tel: 05642-3225

> *Information, counselling and practical assistance and
> treatment on pregnancy and abortion, contraception,
> infertility and psychosexual problems. Well Woman care.
> Fees charged.*

British Infertility Counselling Association
Institute of Obstetrics and Gynaecology
Hammersmith Hospital
Du Cane Road
London wi2 ohs

> *Counselling and advice on the emotional difficulties arising
> from infertility.*

BUPA (British United Provident Association)
Provident House
Essex Street
London WC2R 3AX
Tel: 071-353 9451

> *Private health insurance company that offers screening*
> *programmes.*

Child 'Farthings'
Gaunts Road
Pawlett
Nr Bridgwater
Somerset

> *Support and pressure group on infertility that raises funds*
> *for research. Information and counselling for members.*

Keep Fit Association
16 Upper Woburn Place
London WC1H 0QG

> *Movement training for women of all ages. Leaflets and*
> *addresses of local classes.*

Nuffield Hospitals
Aldwych House
71–91 Aldwych
London WC2B 4EE
Tel: 071-404 0601

PPP (Private Patients Plan)
PPP House
Tunbridge Wells TN1 2PL
Tel: 0892-40111

> *Private health insurance company that offers screening*
> *programmes.*

Ramblers Association
1–4 Crawford Mews
York Street
London W1H 1PT

> *Has town and country branches and organizes walks in the
> company of people of a similar fitness level.*

Sisters Network
c/o Running Magazine
57–61 Mortimer Street
London W1N 7TD

> *Help and encouragement for women wanting to start jogging
> or running. The network will put you in touch with a local
> 'big sister' who will guide and companion you.*

Slimming Magazine Clubs
9 Kendrick Mews
London SW7 3AG
Tel: 071-225 1711

> *See Weight Watchers.*

Sports Council
16 Upper Woburn Place
London WC1H 0QP
Tel: 071-388 1277

> *Can put you in touch with local sports centres and activities.*

Weight Watchers
11 Fairacres
Dedworth Road
Windsor SL4 4UY
Tel: 07538-56751

> *Nationwide network of slimming clubs. Fees charged.*

Index

Page references in italic denote diagrams; es. is used as abbreviation for endometriosis.